Praise for *When Your Adult Child Breaks Your Heart*

"At a time when we have a veritable crisis of adult children coping with mental illness, substance abuse, or their combination—coupled with a lack of resources for their concerned parents—this book provides understandable, practical advice for parents that is useful in real life. Dr. Young is a member of the new generation of psychiatrists unburdened by the tradition of a hierarchy and stereotype and is to be commended for the effort he expended in putting together this concise and practical summary in this important, underserved area. Any parent and clinician would benefit greatly from reading this book."

—David R. Rosenberg, MD, professor and chairman,
Department of Psychiatry and Behavioral Neurosciences,
Wayne State University; and psychiatrist in chief, Detroit Medical Center

"It is often very hard to find help for despairing parents of adult children with mental illness and substance abuse. Easily understood and clearly written, replete with anecdotes, advice, and quotations from real people, this unusually helpful book offers timely and practical information."

—Mark S. Gold, MD, distinguished professor, University of
Florida; and chairman, Department of Psychiatry

"This authoritative guide couples practical, no-nonsense information with support and reassurance. A must-read book for parents who wonder what went wrong and who mistakenly blame themselves."

—Irene S. Levine, PhD, professor of psychiatry,
NYU Langone School of Medicine

WHEN YOUR ADULT CHILD BREAKS YOUR HEART

Coping with Mental Illness, Substance Abuse, and the Problems That Tear Families Apart

JOEL L. YOUNG, MD
AND CHRISTINE ADAMEC

Lyons Press
Guilford, Connecticut
An imprint of Rowman & Littlefield

Lyons Press is an imprint of Rowman & Littlefield.

Distributed by NATIONAL BOOK NETWORK

Library of Congress Cataloging-in-Publication Data is available on file.

ISBN 978-0-7627-9297-9

Printed in the United States of America

The health information expressed in this book is based solely on the personal experience and professional knowledge of the author and is not intended as a medical manual. The information should not be used for diagnosis or treatment, nor as a substitute for professional medical care.

CONTENTS

INTRODUCTION

Most of the time, the struggles of adult children with antisocial personalities, mental illness, or substance abuse fall to their parents and family. The rest of society, wrestling to get by every day with their own concerns, is oblivious to this human drama. Once in a while, these problems stand out in sharp relief, as happened on a winter's morning in Newtown, Connecticut, in 2012. Although we will never be certain what was in the mind of Adam Lanza before he murdered the children and teachers of Sandy Hook Elementary, it became apparent that he was mentally ill. The nation united in grief but divided on solutions. Some people mobilized to ban or limit gun sales, while others focused on the issues of health care accessibility for the mentally ill. Everyone involved in the national conversation became intrigued about Adam's relationship with his mother, the caretaker who spent most of her waking moments with him and who was rewarded with a gunshot wound to the head as she slept.

This book focuses on the parents of adult children with serious issues. Some of these children become violent, although most are not homicidal. Others dispense their anger, depression, and rage on themselves, and spend time teetering on the suicidal brink. Still others harm their own children because their judgment is impaired by mental illness or substances such as alcohol, illegal drugs, or misused prescription drugs. Behind each of these scenes are devastated parents, always laboring about how best to help and uncertain about the coming chaos.

When Your Adult Child Breaks Your Heart is not just a self-help book for parents who are unhappy with their relationships with their adult children. There are a million ways to be disappointed. You may be unhappy that your child did not get through school and has settled on a mediocre job. You might bemoan that he gave up too easily on his athletic career. She might have married someone outside your faith or you might disapprove of how your grandchildren are being raised. These all can be distressing problems, but they have been discussed elsewhere and are not the focus of this volume.

Many of the available books dedicated to the adult child/parent relationship are written *for* adult children who are caring for their elderly parents and who worry about their parents' health and well-being. We reverse the equation. *When Your Adult Child Breaks Your Heart* provides information and advice for parents whose adult children are pushing them to the limits. In this approach, it is the parents of the adult children who are in need of information.

The economic recession of the last few years deeply altered the natural order. The shortage of entry-level jobs and cheap housing forced many adult children to return home. Population researcher Joan R. Kahn identifies this trend in a recent study of shifting economic power between 1960 and 2010. Older Americans are in a stronger financial position than previous senior generations, but the financial strain on younger people is great. She notes, "We find that younger adults have become more financially dependent on their parents and that while older adults have become more financially independent of their adult children, they nevertheless coreside with [live with] their needy adult children."

The researchers found other differences in today's boomerangers. Kahn used census data to demonstrate that even a college education did not immunize a child from returning home. For example, in 1960, of the more than 76,000 adult children living with a parent, only 8.4 percent had a college degree or higher. By 1990, this percentage increased to 16.9 and by 2010, the number of college graduates living with their parents rose to 22.8 percent, a rate nearly three times higher than was observed during the Eisenhower Administration. Needless to say the likelihood of boomeranging increases when an adult child suffers from mental illness or substance abuse or engages in antisocial behaviors or criminal activities.

This book is written for parents whose adult children are actively causing major problems for themselves, their parents, and others. When listening to parents in a therapy office or surveying them online, we learned that there are no limits to the number of ways your children can hurt you. We heard stories about thirty-year-old sons passing out drunk in the local bar and daughters with graduate degrees who regularly shoplift from local stores. Too many parents recount stories of their adult children selling drugs to anyone with money, so that they can buy drugs for themselves. A few parents related instances of their adult children neglecting or physically harming their own young children. We endeavor to understand these inexplicable behaviors and determine that the only answers rest at the nexus between evil behavior and mental illness. Many of the chapters use case studies and current research to explore this relationship further.

It is clear that parents of troubled adult children give up substantial portions of their time, thought, and money to try to help their offspring—often with little to show for their efforts. We hope the book can serve as a resource to help you on this lonely journey. The first chapters examine the meaning of parental responsibility and the physiological impact of this abiding commitment. We raise the question of whether you can only be as happy as your least happy child and leave the issue hotly debated but still unresolved.

You do not need to live with your adult child to worry about him. The psychological effects of coping with your adult child's problems are profound and range from denial to anger and self-blame. The stress can cause changes in appetite and mood. Too often parents blame themselves for the behavior of their adult children, as if they were forever responsible for a child in his thirties or forties. Countering the self-blame misperception is one of our primary missions. Parents need to limit the negative psychological impact in order to help themselves and their families. When you are needlessly overwhelmed and consumed with guilt, it is hard to wipe the kitchen counter let alone tame the beast of your child's mental illness or substance abuse disorder.

Parents need to be strong and well to withstand the barrage that comes with the struggle. Chapter 3 explores the challenge of living under the same roof with your adult child. It concentrates on exasperating situations like watching your child sleep all day and stay up all night. Some parents endure intermittent threats of violence or come to realize that their adult child is stealing or opening the family home to menacing strangers.

Chapter 4 covers the horrific experience of parents whose loved ones abuse their own children. Our criminal justice system comes down hard on violence against children (as it should) and parents of perpetrators have to endure the burden that their child hurt another human being. They also have to adjust to the humiliation of criminal prosecution and the rules that come with incarceration. In jail, adult children are exposed (perhaps yet again) to a lawless culture that values drugs and money over honest work. The friendships an adult forges in prison rarely translate productively after his sentence has been served. Chapter 5 covers issues that are involved when your adult child is accused of or convicted of crimes.

The central truth of our book is that mental illness and substance abuse rest at the core of most problematic behavior. Chapters 6 and 7 define these diagnosable conditions, providing full descriptions of substance use disorders and psychiatric conditions like anxiety disorders, mood disorders, and psychotic disorders. Specific attention is given to ADHD and common personality disorders. Identification and treatment of these underlying conditions is the most efficient way to assist your troubled child.

Suicide is a major risk for substance abusers and the mentally ill. Chapter 8 offers information on the complex behavior of suicide thoughts, attempts, and completions, and outlines ways that parents can help their at-risk children. We follow the worst possible scenario when a child dies by his own hands and how parents carry on after this most brutal act.

Chapter 9 discusses the importance of caring for your own physical and emotional health. Parents often develop deep anxiety and depression necessitating professional treatment, and we offer guidelines for when to seek help. Chapter 10 explores the enormous stress a troubled adult child places on your relationship with your spouse and other adult children. Chapter 11 outlines methods to help your child with personal problem solving. Chapter 12 covers the wrenching situation when you have no choice other than estranging yourself from your child.

This is *not* a fluffy self-help book that will preach to you that all is wonderful and all you need to do is to count your blessings and smile a lot. That wouldn't be realistic or fair. The issues covered within these pages are the tough ones, including substance abuse, mental illness, child abuse, criminal behavior, and suicide. Parents of seriously problematic adult children need this overview, and we hope they benefit from our carefully chosen words and advice.

HOW TO USE THIS BOOK

This book is divided into three major parts, with chapters in each part. You may wish to read each chapter in order until you finish the book, or you may wish to skip ahead to the material that seems the most compelling for you. Part One covers learning to identify and challenge some of your common reactions and mistaken beliefs and ideas. It also includes a chapter on dealing with your problematic adult child when he or she lives with you. We recommend you read this chapter even if your adult child does *not* live with you, because it includes many valuable tips for dealing with anger and aggression.

The chapters in Part Two offer specific examples of problematic behavior, such as the adult child with a substance abuse issue or mental illness who mistreats his children. Other chapters cover adult children who commit crimes, issues of substance abuse, psychiatric diagnoses that may be the key cause of behavioral problems, and suicidal behaviors that may occur in an adult child.

Each chapter discusses ways that you may be able to help your adult children, as well as situations in which you likely need to back off. In some cases, you may even need to take action *against* your adult child, which is particularly hard. For example, if your daughter is abusing alcohol and leaving your two-year-old grandson alone or with disreputable people, you will need to make tough decisions. Certainly your first action is to protect your grandchild. Then what? Simply hope for her to stop drinking? You may also need to call the child protective services authorities to report the neglect. This will force an investigation, which might result in the removal of the child from your daughter's home. This is not an easy action to take for any parent of an adult child! This book is not about easy answers, but about facing the tough realities emanating from your adult child's behavior, and managing them as best as you can—without sacrificing yourself in the process.

Part Three covers ways to care for yourself while your adult child is exhibiting problematic behavior. In some cases, your distress over the child's problematic behavior may have propelled you into a state of clinical depression. The best way of caring for your family is by caring for yourself first.

One definition of insanity is to keep doing the same thing repeatedly, while each time expecting a different result. Yet this is what many parents of problematic adult children do—they give them money (sometimes a *lot* of money), they internalize the adult child's verbal abuse, and they spend too much time agonizing over the adult child's troubles. This book offers suggestions on how to stop these behaviors.

Also in Part Three are methods to resolve your concerns with your adult child in a realistic way, including talking about the limitations of the help you can and will provide. Parents of adult children who abuse drugs, mistreat family members, and cheat and lie may have to make the painful decision to walk away from their child until he decides to get help or to change his ways. Sometimes the best decision for a parent is simply to withdraw, and we offer criteria on how to know if that is the best decision available to you.

This book is based on the latest research and interspersed with many case studies. We have seen many bleak situations improve, but we discourage the destructive kind of hope that is based on magical thinking—that someday the bad behavior of the adult child will cease and the person you really want him to be will emerge from the swampy fog to happily rejoin everyday society. It *can* happen, and sometimes does, but such spontaneous occurrences are unlikely. At the end, getting from "there" to "here" requires parents to possess finesse and discipline and the humility to recognize that these traits are dwarfed in importance if your child is not ready to make the necessary changes.

NOTE TO READERS

At the beginning of many chapters, we provide a direct quotation from an unidentified parent of an adult child with serious issues. These quotations were derived from individuals who responded to our survey questionnaire and from actual patients. We took appropriate license to alter the details to protect privacy. Some chapters begin with or later offer case study information, and again we protected the identity of the individuals.

PART ONE

IDENTIFYING THE PROBLEMS

Part One describes important issues such as your role as a parent when your children are grown and how responsible you are (or are not) for them. It also covers your emotional reactions when your adult child experiences difficult issues. Finally, this part discusses problems that may come up when your adult child lives with you and offers active coping suggestions.

CHAPTER 1

UNDERSTANDING THE SEVERE PROBLEMS ADULT CHILDREN CAN CAUSE

My son is now twenty-eight years old, but the serious problems and the abuse started in his teenage years. On many occasions, he has been very physically abusive to me. At different times, he has pinned me to the floor by my neck, swung a skateboard right at my head, and twisted my arm behind my back so hard that I thought that he would dislocate it. Then he started attacking his brother, but he was big enough to defend himself and his brother fought back.

Doctors have diagnosed my son with depression and borderline personality disorder, and he also has a problem with drugs.

When Adam Lanza opened fire and killed twenty children and six adults at the Sandy Hook Elementary School in Newtown, Connecticut, the massacre shattered the lives of countless families and wounded the entire nation.

Thankfully, tragedies of this magnitude are rare in American life, but the incident at Newtown did allow the national conversation to explore the relationship of mental illness and violence and the burden of raising a child with severe mental health problems.

Behind nearly every adult who is mentally ill, or who becomes addicted to drugs or alcohol, or who neglects or abuses their children, or who commits a serious crime, there is a suffering parent. This parent may initially react to the news of his or her adult child's behavior with horror, anger, and a natural desire to rectify the situation.

These immediate reactions are then rapidly followed by major emotional doubts and fears, such as, "What did I do wrong when he was a child to make him act this way now? Was it something I said or did? Or was it something that I *failed* to do years ago? Is this really somehow all *my* fault?" Had Nancy Lanza been spared by her son Adam, she would undoubtedly have suffered self-recriminations and wondered where she went wrong. (Certainly one major mistake that she *did* make was in maintaining firearms at her home. No parent of a mentally ill child should ever provide access to guns.)

For many parents, helping their child is an all-consuming task. They open their pocketbooks, empty their IRAs, and let their adult children move back home. These parents put their lives on hold (vacations, retirement, hopes, and dreams) in order to guide their children away from yet another disaster. They devote astonishing efforts to one overriding mission: to help their adult child.

Yet in most cases, only the adult children can make the major decisions: whether to take their psychiatric medicines, engage in meaningful therapy, get a job, attend Alcoholics Anonymous, or take other actions to solve their problems.

PARENTS FOR YOUR WHOLE LIFE?

Parents of adult children with serious problems will frequently risk their own physical, emotional, and financial health in extreme attempts to resolve the problems that are caused by their adult children's issues. For most parents, there is no statute of limitations on helping your child and instead, their impulse is to respond to their child's needs whether that child is ten or thirty.

"I have to help my daughter," they may tell themselves. "She really needs me now." Or, "My son is in trouble and no one else will help him like me. I must come to the rescue."

Pop psychology has a demeaning name for parents and spouses of the mentally ill: enablers. Put another way, these are individuals who unknowingly perpetuate the existing problems of the adult child through their own behavior. When used accurately, the term "enablers" refers to a specific population, such as parents who continue to supply alcohol to their son with liver cirrhosis caused by drinking. But when loosely used, the term has come to imply that families are responsible for their child's mental illness, and that they somehow encourage anxiety, depression, and substance misuse. This perverse logic holds that families control the on/off switch of their child's behaviors.

A MOTHER'S PLEA

Shortly after Newtown, a woman named Liza Long wrote an essay for an online site that soon went viral. Titled, "I Am Adam Lanza's Mother," it begged for a robust discussion on mental illness. In it Long described her daily routine with her thirteen-year-old mentally ill son. She described how his sweet sensibility was replaced unpredictably by intense temper tantrums. With each passing day, she saw him become stronger and more fearless. She knew that soon she would no longer be able to contain him and protect her other children from his impulsive outbursts. Liza Long both loved and feared her child and she felt alone in the struggle.

Long was praised by supporters but vilified by others for "outing" her son's mental illness and exposing him to potential embarrassment. Others argued that parents alone are responsible for their child's behavior and stated their view that her son's mild autism spectrum disorder (formerly known as Asperger's syndrome) and ADHD were not legitimate illnesses. They judged Long to be an inadequate mother. In response, many pointed out that if she had written about a child with cancer or some other nonstigmatized disease, she would have drawn universal sympathy. Long's essay and the heated debate it spawned underscored that in the second decade of this century, mental illness may no longer be in the closet, but it is still not well understood.

Liza Long's essay was courageous and motivated by an interest in opening a dialogue over the difficulties that parents face with their mentally ill children. At the core of this conversation are the facts. Most mentally ill people do not harm or murder innocent people. Many live among us and lead quiet and productive lives far from the headlines of cable news and the Internet. Yet we cannot minimize other truths. The severely mentally ill are overrepresented in the criminal justice system. Psychiatric issues do contribute to many sensationalistic stories. Mental illness often starts in childhood and persists into adulthood, and is associated with undereducation, underemployment, and family strife. Parents of adult children are often left to cope with the daily struggles on their own. Long's essay argues that the effects of mental illness on the family are too risky for American society to ignore. The sooner we acknowledge this, the faster we can respond to the great need.

If you are reading this book because your child is breaking your heart, take a step back to reflect. Do you remember what awful thing you did to your child to make him exhibit bad behavior as an adult? Are you in any way—physically, emotionally, or financially—benefiting from your child's illness? We doubt the answer is yes. Chances are you did nothing to harm your children and instead, you tried as hard as you could to help them.

In the aftermath of a publicized tragedy or in the conversations of daily life, it is a common reflex of media as well as the general public to blame parents for their child's behavior. This underlying current of disapproval, particularly when it is shared by friends and family, adds to the heavy burden that these parents are already facing. Yet in opposition to the all-out sprint to demonize Nancy Lanza for her youngest son's actions is the fact that the Lanzas' older son is a successful accountant and a well-respected member of his community. Unless they themselves are psychotic, parents do not choose one child to do well and the other to fail; they do not enable their child to commit destruction. Rather, they earnestly raise them as best they can.

Being labeled an enabler is usually the least of a parent's problems. Most families of troubled adult children face constant anxiety as a result of their loved one's unpredictable and uncontrollable behavior. These parents are psychologically traumatized by their previous encounters with the police or courts, and when sensing new problems, their anxiety can cascade into panic and depression. When trouble comes again, they mobilize all their resources, not just to protect their children, but also to maintain their own emotional health. The toll of repeated trauma and anxiety is incalculable.

Children Affect Their Parents—For Life

Your children are yours from the day they are born to the day you die. Your impact on them lingers after you are gone. Entire developmental psychology books explore parents' influence on their young. But what is left out of most books—what most parents already know—is that the reverse is true as well: Children affect their parents.

In a recent study published in 2006 in the *Journal of Marriage and the Family*, Emily A. Greenfield and Nadine F. Marks queried the parents about their adult children's overall functioning. The researchers tallied emotional, financial, and substance abuse problems as well as the adult children's employment and marital status. They found that the greater number of problems that their adult children had experienced, the lower was the parents' positive affect (happiness). Problems of adult children also led to a lower level of parental self-acceptance and to greater family relationship strain.

Other scholars have made inroads into long-unchallenged theories about parents and their children. Anne-Marie Ambert's findings in her book *The Effect of Children on Parents* disrupted the established order of family systems theory, which assumed that the impact could only be top-down (the parents' effects on their children). Ambert concluded that the traditional top-down model has misled large numbers of parents and professionals into believing that parents largely control their children. Thus, when children actively misbehave in public, the generally accepted belief is that their parents must have failed them in some way, that they must be "bad parents." Many parents internalize this notion as well, often unfairly.

So if the parents' impact on their children is finite, what causes things to go wrong? To be fair, Ambert acknowledged that some parents are ineffective or worse. No one can deny that children abandoned by their fathers or raised without physical nurturing are at a disadvantage compared to their peers. Such factors are clearly responsible for some children's problematic behavior. But Ambert also observed that social groups, peer groups, and others can also powerfully impact a child's well-being and his transformation into adulthood.

External Impacts on Psychological Development

Your child is exposed to endless situations and conflicts as he journeys through childhood and into adolescence and then adulthood, and many of these experiences ultimately impact whom he becomes. Once a child leaves the realm of the parental home, whether it be to early day care at the age of six weeks or to kindergarten at age five, he is constantly bombarded with the behaviors of others, to which he must respond or withdraw. For example, if natural male aggression in little boys is discouraged by the family, the child will temper his inclinations or risk isolation from mostly female caregivers and teachers. But if aggression is overly valued in his outside world, as in the world of street gangs, then that aggression will be ratcheted up in a direct response to what the peer group expects.

Teachers, pediatricians, and parents must be astute to pick up on warning signs of these external influences. Consider the role of bullying by one's peers. Bullying can begin in the earliest grades and it often goes undetected. To be bullied means that every day the child faces shame. Recent understanding of bullying links it to the victim acting out and even to teenage suicide. The impact of a lifetime of bullying persists into adulthood and the separation of time and distance from the experience is only partially healing.

Failure in school will also have an impact on the child into adulthood. Not uncommonly, undiagnosed ADHD or a learning disability can account for a child's struggles. All too frequently these conditions are missed and proper treatment is not given. For the child, school becomes an exercise in futility and begins a path through life with a negative and distorted self-perception. As with bullying, the humiliation lasts a lifetime.

Other social factors impact the developing mind. For example, if as a parent you consistently stressed the virtue of honesty to your children, but they later learn that they must cheat in order to survive at school, they may, despite presumably deeply learned moral values, succumb to the lure. Survival and success become more valued traits than being "good."

While we cannot break down the impact that each of these factors has on how our children turn out, it is clear that direct parenting is not the total story. This is why we chose to write this book. We want to encourage parents to avoid taking responsibility for all their adult child's missteps and stop attributing a child's problems to some mysterious error that was made during her childhood. When things go awry, it is natural to blame someone, and unfortunately parents, particularly mothers, have historically been the target. It's time to move away from this idea.

If you can't think what terrible thing you did to doom your adult child, then you probably didn't do any terrible thing at all. It is more accurate to blame their behavior on mental illness and addiction or medical disorders that are outside your control. This perspective, supported by the bulk of contemporary research, advances the conclusion that parents have limited control over their children. Sometimes bad things happen to the ones we love the most, and we just don't know why. Much of our book examines the link between mental illness and substance abuse and the consequent problems of adult children. We describe the common psychiatric disorders affecting adult children and attempt to get a handle on the available medications and therapies. We never lose sight that the medical management of these conditions, as with parenting, is limited.

A Continued Link

Parents are inextricably linked to their children. A number of things account for this connection, including basic pride. Attributing the success or failure of children to their parents is so ingrained that the momentum for blaming or crediting parents carries into adulthood. On this level, parents are invested in their children's success because it directly reflects on them, what is termed as their core competency. Social biologists do not disagree. The natural desire for parents to want their offspring to do well in life, to "make them proud," may reflect an instinctive drive for immortality. Living creatures have a self-interest in perpetuating their own genes; this instinct is at the foundation of reproduction. If children fail to position themselves for reproductive success as they sometimes do, parents respond by helping their adult child make a life course correction. Increasing evidence suggests that this connection is hardwired into the brain.

ARE YOU ONLY AS HAPPY AS YOUR LEAST HAPPY CHILD?

Are you only as happy as your least happy adult child? Some parents agree, and there is research to back it up. For example, in 2011, a study by Karen Fingerman and her colleagues reported in the *Journal of Gerontology* on 633 middle-aged parents who had 1,384 grown children. The researchers had the parents evaluate their children on two scales. The first scale measured physical and emotional problems, such as developmental delays, psychological problems, health issues, and physical disabilities. The second scale measured lifestyle and behavioral problems, which included drinking and drug problems, as well as legal and financial issues. The parents were then asked to rate their adult children in terms of the children's failures or successes.

In single child families, 43 percent reported problems with their child. However, in families with two children, more than two-thirds had at least one adult child with a problem. In families with three adult children the risk that at least one child had a problem was 83 percent.

Overall, more than two-thirds of the parents reported that their child had at least one problem within the past two years. These parents also reported a diminished sense of their own personal well-being. About half of the parents rated their children to be above average in success, but that factor alone did not predict parental well-being. If one child of a family with multiple children was having problems, even as his siblings were thriving, their parents were negatively affected. Indeed the research confirms that an adult child's problems seemed contagious and that parents only seemed as happy as their least happy child. Even among parents who reported having their own serious problems, the successes or problems of their adult children significantly affected the well-being of their parents. As discussed in chapter 10, successful children are also affected, as they come to resent that their troubled siblings dominate their parents' ability to find joy.

Does it really have to be this way? Certainly, parents will become upset if their adult children are unhappy. But at the same time, ceding control of your personal happiness to someone else, even someone you love as much as your children, is a strategy that allows them too much power over you. This book offers parents many ways to understand their troubled adult child. This includes insight into the illnesses that explain their behavior and proper ways to combat these illnesses. We realize that sometimes the best intervention does not improve the outcome and you may need to confront this possibility. In some cases, parents need to be prepared to walk away and become estranged.

ADULT CHILDREN AND SUBSTANCE ABUSE

The abuse of alcohol and/or drugs is a major problem among adults, whose parents then worry about their risk for being involved in accidents, for neglecting their children, and harming their partners. They are also at higher risk for suicide. We cover more about substance abuse in chapter 6; this is an overview.

Alcohol Abuse and Alcoholism

In 2010, more than two-thirds of all American adults consumed alcohol, and alcohol consumption itself is on the rise in the United States. Of course, not everyone who consumes alcohol has a substance abuse diagnosis, but a dramatically higher rate reflects a nationwide problem. Excessive alcohol consumption is indicative of large numbers of unhappy individuals who are finding a way, albeit a destructive way, to feel better. Some of them are adult children whose parents are trying, often in vain, to help them. Some also have to deal with binge drinking, a particularly dangerous way of consuming alcohol. Defined as consuming five or more drinks at one time for men or four or more drinks at one time for women, this behavior increases the risk of alcohol poisoning, a potentially fatal condition in which the liver cannot process the high levels of alcohol in the system. Death can result if alcohol poisoning is unidentified and untreated (perhaps because others think that the person is just "sleeping it off").

Drug Abuse and Addiction

Some adults are deeply involved in the abuse and/or the selling of illegal drugs or misappropriated prescription drugs. While the number of drug arrests for juveniles (under age eighteen) has remained pretty flat over the period 1970–2007, the arrests among adults for the use and abuse of drugs have skyrocketed, according to the FBI's Bureau of Justice Statistics.

Some adults abuse illegal drugs, such as marijuana or methamphetamine, while others abuse prescribed prescription painkillers (oxycodone, hydrocodone, and other prescribed drugs). Other individuals abuse controlled psychotherapeutic drugs, such as Xanax (alprazolam) or stimulants such as Adderall (mixed amphetamine salts).

FATHERS WITH ADULT CHILDREN WHO ARE MENTALLY ILL

Mothers bear the brunt of their children's illness, but fathers are not immune. A small but illuminating study of ten fathers of mentally ill adults was published in *Issues in Mental Health Nursing* in 2012. The adult children had various psychiatric conditions ranging from obsessive-compulsive disorder (OCD) to schizophrenia and depression. Some of the fathers felt exhausted by their ongoing uncertainty about their children. The fathers said they were generally relegated to passive tasks, like observing their children's level of activity and aggression and other signs of deteriorating mental health. One father ate lunch with his child daily so he could monitor his adult child's behavior.

Many of the fathers in the study identified their own sense of powerlessness over their child's plight. One father, a victim of his son's knife attack, lamented that he had to turn to law enforcement authorities as a last resort to get help for his child. Another shuddered about his daughter's multiple suicide attempts. After one serious overdose, he was told by a doctor that she might not survive. She did survive, but years later the memory still haunts him.

Interestingly, most of the fathers surveyed believed that mothers still carried the heavier burden. But the fathers of mentally ill children often do suffer, and their suffering is considerable.

Substance Abuse and Crime

Parents of substance abusing adult children always worry about the next crisis. The need to buy illegal drugs fuels much criminal behavior, some of which occurs among adult children. More than one family has scoured the local pawnshops to buy back stolen keepsakes. It is a painful realization to know that if your adult child is stealing from you, then he is probably stealing from others too.

The troubles that accompany substance abuse are limitless and their families bear witness to the consequences. Drunk driving continues to kill thousands of Americans yearly, and behind nearly all perpetrators is a suffering family. Drugged individuals are also more likely to commit crimes.

Substance abusers with minor children are more likely to abuse or neglect their own children. Alcohol intoxications are associated with violent outbursts, leaving nobody safe in the household. Methamphetamine abusers may be abusive or may ignore their young children altogether. They may fall asleep while their children roam free and unsupervised. Read more about child abuse in chapter 4, criminal behavior in chapter 5, and substance abuse in chapter 6.

Money Issues and Substance Abuse

Money becomes a major concern for many parents of troubled adult children. Most parents hope that their last major financial obligation for their child is paying for college tuition and textbook money. It is downright disheartening to pay for bail and legal services, or worse.

Paul was a thirty-seven-year-old banker who was accused of assaulting his wife. He implored his parents to lend him the money to retain an expensive private attorney. At first, his parents funded the request—or so they thought. The money was actually diverted by Paul to purchase oxycodone off the streets. His stated need for a private attorney was just an excuse to fund his drug habit.

Once the pattern of lying became clearly and painfully apparent, Paul's parents came to the uncomfortable understanding that their substance-dependent child could and would lie to them in the service of his own addiction. For an addict, there are really only two important goals in life. One is using the drug and the other is figuring out how to obtain more of it.

MENTAL ILLNESS

Some adult children develop psychiatric disorders for the first time in adulthood, while in other cases, the illness first appears in childhood or adolescence and remains a problem for the person throughout their lives. Of course, having a psychiatric disorder doesn't mean someone is "bad," although mental illness is still stigmatized in our society, particularly severe mental illness. But if adult children are also abusing substances and stealing or attacking others, these behaviors *are* very problematic for their parents and others in society. In addition, the symptoms of mental illness can be very difficult for parents to deal with, as when the child is experiencing hallucinations, has delusions of persecution, or has fixed false beliefs that their parents are actively plotting against them. (Read more in chapter 3 about how to deal with such symptoms.)

In chapter 7, we describe in greater detail common psychiatric conditions such as severe depression or anxiety disorders, bipolar disorder, severe adult attention-deficit hyperactivity disorder (ADHD), and some personality disorders, such as borderline personality disorder and antisocial personality disorder. Often people with psychiatric problems have two or more disorders. Psychiatrists refer to this as having "comorbidities," a technical term that sounds as if a person were simultaneously dying from two or more diseases. But what it generally means is that the disorders are treated in sequence, the more severe one first, followed by treatment of the next one, and then treatment for any other psychiatric issues.

As an example, an adult suffering from severe depression may also have an impairing level of ADHD, while an individual with schizophrenia may also have an antisocial personality disorder. Usually one psychiatric condition is considered as dominant, but the treatment team actively works to resolve both (or all, if more than two problems exist). Patients with two or more psychiatric conditions are more challenging to treat and they also generally have a less favorable outcome.

Parents of adults with psychiatric disorders usually know they cannot cure them, but by better understanding the possible root causes they can also learn the best means to obtain psychiatric help. Sadly, the ultimate choices for the lives of the mentally ill adult children, no matter how impaired they are, almost always lie with the adult child. This is a very tough lesson for parents to learn, and some people never learn it. We hope that our readers use our strategies and examples to help their children and themselves, but also that they do not believe there are any magical fixes for the problems we describe.

COMMON MISTAKEN BELIEFS

Many parents of adult children with serious issues hold common flawed beliefs, including the following examples:

- If I try hard enough, then I can help my adult child fix this problem (and conversely, if she doesn't get better, I wasn't trying hard enough).
- I must sacrifice to support my adult child.
- No one in our family or among our friends has ever done this bad thing before (gone to jail/used drugs, and so forth).
- If my child truly loved me, then he would not act this way.

Common Belief: If I Try Hard Enough, I Can Fix This

Many people are accustomed to thinking that they can solve just about any problem with a good plan and focused effort. Recalcitrant adult children can stymie that belief. The truth is no one will change if they do not feel the need to change. Sure, there are steps you can take to help sway them, such as connecting an alcoholic child to Alcoholics Anonymous or urging a depressed child to seek psychiatric help. You can make the case for change, but the final decision remains out of your hands.

However, there are times that you can force treatment. All states provide for involuntary commitment if a mentally ill person demonstrates that he is an imminent threat to himself or others. An example would be a psychotic individual experiencing command hallucinations demanding that he kill a police officer. Involuntary commitment is a civil procedure when the patient is remanded to a psychiatric hospital for a brief time by court order. The law generally distinguishes psychiatric conditions from substance use disorders. For instance, if threats are made when the individual is high or intoxicated, states generally do not allow involuntary commitment. Conversely, if your adult child commits a crime, the court may step in and order psychiatric treatment.

This acceptance of your own limited powers over your mentally ill adult child may take years to achieve and is often hard-won. Once you can take this step, it can bring an enormous sense of relief.

Common Belief: I Must Sacrifice to Help My Adult Child

Some parents delay their retirement or postpone long-awaited vacations to help their troubled adult children. It is easy to rationalize delayed gratification with such statements as, "How can I enjoy myself or how can we spend money on ourselves when our child is failing so miserably?"

This act of selflessness may not be shared by your spouse or appreciated by your troubled child. The decision of how much money parents should donate to their child's cause is a delicate negotiation shaped by the extent of your child's problems and your own financial situation. Be careful not to go through your own savings or max out your credit cards in this effort. If you've already started down this path, then stop now. When faced with the dilemma of adult children with serious issues, parents experience spiritual heartbreak and tough financial decisions, both of which have the potential to tear apart the heartiest marriage.

Common Belief: This Doesn't Happen to My Friends and I Don't Know Whom to Trust

When your adult child gets arrested for driving under the influence of alcohol (DUI), goes to jail, or commits other offensive behaviors, you are liable to feel quite isolated. You may think that no one in your social sphere has endured the experience. You may be right, but you probably aren't. Bad behavior is fairly common among adult children, but most families fear being exposed to gossip and shame. When bad things happen, parents have to balance the comfort they derive from receiving solace from friends and family with the risk of exposing too much. Two examples illuminate this precarious choice:

Mona recalls having lunch with two friends when she disclosed that her twenty-five-year-old daughter had just been arrested for selling marijuana. She was surprised when Anita, her friend since childhood, broke the shocked silence. "I told you that Donny went out of state to get a great job. But I lied to you. He's really in prison for five years for assaulting his ex-girlfriend." There is shared comfort in misery and both women gently winced at their collective misfortune. They were both furious, however, when they learned weeks later that their private exchange had become public knowledge. Apparently the third woman at the table felt the disclosure was too juicy to resist and launched it into the local gossip circuit.

Trusting conversations do not always become acts of betrayal. Carrie was surprised to meet a casual friend in the waiting area of the state prison two hundred miles from her home. For years, both women had served side by side on a church committee. Until their fateful meeting, neither could have ever imagined that the other had an imprisoned son. Their shared experience solidified their friendship and gave them sustained comfort. Such events underscore that none of us completely knows what is happening in the homes and families of our friends and neighbors.

Common Belief: If My Child Truly Loved Me, He Would Not Act This Way

Faced with unrelenting bad news, it's hard to decipher your adult child's motivation. It is natural to equate his actions with a sense that he no longer loves you. It is true that in a drug-addled state, or in the throes of a psychotic break, it may be unclear to him whom he loves, but parents need to remember that losing a child's love is an uncommon occurrence.

In most cases, your adult child's behavior is really not about you at all. Instead, it's about her addiction or mental illness. The effects of drugs and alcohol account for the bad actions of otherwise good people. Adult children with extreme social anxiety or obsessive-compulsive disorder don't get jobs because of their intense fears, and not because they want to punish their parents for some long lapsed misdeed. Individuals with ADHD act rashly because they are uncontrollably impulsive, not because they have contempt for you. Still, in dire circumstances it is hard to acknowledge that your child's love offers little immunization from bearing great pain. These concepts are further developed in the next few chapters.

DIFFERENT TYPES OF STRUGGLING PARENTS

Parents of troubled adult children are as diverse as are their children's problems. Children with ADHD can be born to lesbian parents and schizophrenia can invade the world of staid college professors. Antisocial children can be raised by Army brass or immigrant tailors. Parents can be young or old, fortunate to have adequate means or struggling from one paycheck to the next. Despite the endless combinations, certain categories emerge to describe how parents cope. You may recognize yourself in one or more of these descriptions. If not, do not despair. You will no doubt find yourself in some of the cases that are offered in the succeeding chapters.

The Fixer/Problem-Solver

Some parents have a natural instinct to fix the problems that their child creates. This resourcefulness can be essential; for instance, the skill to find a good doctor or treatment facility can help save your child.

Therapists and psychiatrists like working with fixers. Fixers are usually analytical and logical, and they understand cause and effect. Fixers readily understand that an adult child with a mental illness will function considerably better when they follow the doctor's orders. For example, medication noncompliance (refusing to take their medicine) in bipolar disorder can unleash full mania, characterized by spending money wildly, engaging in unprotected sex with inappropriate people, and other unpredictable behaviors. Mood-stabilizing medications can treat current manic episodes and prevent further ones from developing.

Fixers efficiently find methods to improve their bipolar child's medication compliance. They are open to the suggestions of their treatment team and usually are one step ahead with devising a good plan even if the adult children themselves are not yet ready for help. The problem lies when your child rejects your solutions. For the fixer, this can be very difficult to understand. It seems logical that a person with a drug or alcohol problem *should* go to rehab. It is infuriating for the fixer when his child is unwilling or unready to receive such treatment.

The Rescuer

The rescuer may be akin to the fixer, in that they are willing to swoop in to save the adult child from any and all problems. But the rescuer may be more ardent and emotional than the fixer, and thus will become more distressed when her solutions are ignored.

Rescuers act from the heart and become so invested in their children's woes that they can put their own lives on hold until their child's issues are resolved. They are eager to help their children but may go about it inefficiently. Rescuers may throw money at a problem, but they are less committed to a specific course of action.

Lilly's parents exemplify the patterns of rescuers. They were deeply frustrated by Lilly's run-ins with the police due to her chronic shoplifting. But rather than encouraging her to stay focused on her psychotherapy and to be compliant with taking her OCD and ADHD medications, the family instead bitterly blamed Lilly's doctors. In their zeal to rescue her, they wasted time and resources to duplicate the identical treatment plan with a different team. They were rescuing her—but from the wrong threat.

The Self-Blamer

As mentioned earlier, some parents blame themselves for all the serious problems that their children encounter. But self-blaming is a recipe for poor physical and mental health, including the development of hypertension and depression. (Read more about taking care of your own health in chapter 9.) Consider this: Thinking that you are to derive all credit or blame for your child's life is grandiose. How could anyone other than the individual really have that much power?

Don't shortchange yourself and others in your family by agonizing over what you did or could have done to cause your adult child to behave as he does now. Avoid the very common "woulda, coulda, shoulda" mentality. Remember, you are not omnipotent, and in part, your child is the product of the prevailing culture and the influences of his peers and co-workers.

Self-blamers often struggle with their own mental health. This is explained on two levels. First, mood disorders, substance dependency, and ADHD tend to run in families. You may not have caused your adult child's particular problems, but it is possible that he may have inherited from you a genetic predisposition for a psychiatric illness.

Secondly, guilt and repetitive negative thoughts are often symptoms of depression, and if you or your spouse is depressed (or sometimes both

---

AN EXERCISE FOR THE SELF-BLAMER

If you are a self-blamer, the following exercise can be useful.

First, are you responsible for wars that occur throughout the world? You're not? Okay.

What about the state of the economy. Are you personally responsible for the price of gas and for the unemployment rate? No? That's right, you're not! Even the president of the United States can't easily manipulate these items, although he has far more power than you do.

Think about your entire extended family, including aunts, uncles, cousins, grandparents, in-laws, the whole lot, except for your own children. Is anyone in this group unhappy or miserable? It's pretty likely that at least a few of them *are* unhappy. If so, is it your fault? If not you, then whose fault is it?

Now move into considering your own adult children, and think about the problems that they may have now. Did you make them abuse drugs or alcohol? Did you put a curse on them and somehow cause them to have a mental illness? You didn't, did you?

Accept responsibility for what *is* your fault (although do not agonize over it endlessly), while at the same time, identify where your sphere of influence lies and where it ends. It is likely far narrower than you ever imagined.

---

of you become depressed), then you're more likely to feel guilt and blame yourself for your adult child's problems and issues. Seek your own treatment to disentangle these emotions and to fortify yourselves to best help your children.

The Codependent

The codependent parent is enmeshed in the life of her adult child and cannot distinguish between serving her child and doing right by him. Codependent parents buy beer for their alcoholic son or hide his empty bottles from their spouse. They call their daughter's work when she is too hung over to wake up and tell her boss that she has food poisoning and can't come in.

Codependency is associated with the families of substance abusers, but the behavior is not limited to this population. Codependent parents continue to pay for their child's excessive shopping bills. They cover their fully employed son's gambling debts and look the other way when he neglects to pay his child support. They purchase term papers off the Internet when their college junior forgets to write her English assignment.

Codependency is problematic for both parties, as it locks parents and their children into a negative and nonproductive relationship. Protecting an adult from the consequences of her actions, even as her parents believe that they are doing right, is highly misguided behavior.

Codependent individuals often respond well to both individual and group therapy. Many times, parents are unaware of their own behavior and its consequences, and an objective third party (an honest therapist or the other members of a peer support group) can serve as a mirror to help the codependent person identify and then reverse recurrent problematic patterns.

The Helpless Person

Some people feel that they are unable to combat any of their adult child's problematic behavior. Shari recalls a terrifying experience. "My son went through a phase when he brought strangers into our basement. He thought they were innocent friends to get high with. I was terrified and did not know what to do."

In this book, we offer techniques to assist the helpless person regain her life from her dominating children. The most important lesson is the truth. You need to break out of your passivity, for your own safety and well-being. If you let your child bring frightening people into your home because you feel helpless, you will feel far worse one day when your son's "friends" break into your house to steal valuables that they scoped out when they were guests, or when the SWAT team breaks down your front door to search your house for drugs.

Helpless people feel hopeless, and those who lose hope cannot solve problems.

KEY POINTS IN THIS CHAPTER

- Many people think that if your children of any age have a serious problem, then it is your fault because you were undoubtedly a bad parent. Often they are wrong.

- Parents may be only as happy as their least happy adult child—but it doesn't have to be this way.

- Parents of adults who have serious issues may have common misguided beliefs, such as that they must provide all the financial help that their children ever may need.

- Unhappy parents of distressed children may fall into several categories: the fixer, the enabler, the helpless person, the codependent, and the rescuer. Learning your type will help liberate you.

The next chapter covers common emotional and behavioral issues and misconceptions that parents of adult children with serious issues must face. Read this chapter carefully and see if you recognize yourself or someone else whom you know in the examples that are provided.

CHAPTER 2
YOUR EMOTIONS AND BEHAVIORAL REACTIONS

My thirty-five-year-old daughter doesn't have a formal diagnosis, but she has been picked up by the police at least twice from bars after becoming totally belligerent. They have taken her to jail twice to sleep it off. She has also lost jobs because of going out to lunch drinking and then never getting back to work. It's very frustrating to see her do stuff like this, over and over.

For most parents of adult children whose behavior severely deteriorates, whether they are in trouble with the law, drinking too much, or ignoring their own children, it's often very hard *not* to flash back to an image of your child when he was a sweet little three-year-old. He had such big eyes and soft hair, as he trustingly gazed up at you and asked you to hold his hand so you could go for a walk around the block together.

Or maybe you have an image of when your third grader won an art contest for the most beautiful drawing in her elementary school. She was so precious and creative—the fact that she was a little louder and a little more spontaneous than her friends made her even more wonderful to you.

So how on earth did your child morph into this adult monster, a person who punches holes in the drywall, screams obscenities at you, and mistreats his own wife and children? Or into your son who won't get a job and stares lifelessly at the television? Is he even hearing or seeing the images in front of him? You can't really tell. Or maybe your daughter is abusing substances, although you aren't really sure if it's street drugs or prescription medications. You conclude that it's probably both.

Many children go through difficult periods, and either through the blessings of time or active treatment, they eventually overcome their demons. The universal redemption for parents is to witness your child overcoming his obstacles, whether this involves a stutter or a struggle with

HE CALLS: MY HEART SINKS

Every time the phone rings, and I see that it's my son, I have a sinking feeling right in the pit of my stomach. I know it's going to be a fight over money, and that he usually wins. I have no savings now, and I have overdrawn on my checking account several times because I have given him money that I really didn't have but that he needed. How can I say no to my own son if he really needs my help?

weight. If your child has captured that sweet success, you are probably not reading this book. We have written this book for less fortunate parents who dream for better things.

In many cases, nothing you have done to persuade your adult child, from reasoning to pleading to bribing, has worked. No matter what you try, and no matter how hard you try, you can't get through to him. He has built a stone wall of psychological defenses that you just cannot penetrate. You may think you simply haven't found the one right thing to say, but in most cases, the problem is not your failure to communicate.

The underlying problem is often that you can't "fix" him because he is not ready to be fixed. It is more than likely that he does not share your perception that things have gone awry. He may refuse to enter rehab, seek professional help, or do anything to improve the current debacle that is his life. At times you might succeed temporarily; your child might demonstrate moments of insight that give you hope. But too often, he returns to the same past self-defeating behavior. This is the cycle of hope and disappointment that is so well known to many parents of troubled adult children.

Is that little girl you remember so vividly still inside this raging adult who is violating so many of your values? Of course she is, although her innocence is pretty well camouflaged right now. The reality, however, is that in her current state she is really *not* a person whom you would ever want to know if she were not your child. That's tough to write, or to read.

Your adult child's poor choices can cut you to the core. Parents can feel panicked, sad, helpless, and humiliated. You may also start to lash out with irritability and may isolate yourself from your friends. It is easy to become consumed with thoughts about your children, and this preoccupation can suffocate other important family relationships. This chapter explores the emotional reactions and behavioral tendencies of parents at the brink.

SHE ACTS: YOU REACT

When parents of adult children initially discover their children's seriously problematic behaviors, they often have major emotional reactions, including disbelief and shock (my child couldn't possibly have done *this*!), guilt and self-blame, and anger. If the transgression is new, there is a natural reaction to align with your child, loyally and blindly coming to her defense.

Many times these problem patterns keep recurring. One wonders if Yogi Berra was addressing a group of parents of adult children with issues when he observed, "It's déjà vu, all over again." The emergence of these familiar emotions can quickly negate what was previously a happy day for you. See if you can relate to any of these reactions:

- Denial and shock
- Guilt and self-blame
- Anger
- Anxiety and depression

AN ANGRY TEENAGE SON BECOMES
AN ANGRY ADULT MALE

My son can be abusive, and he screams and throws things. This first happened when he was a child and he's still doing it at age twenty-five. Back when he was a teenager, he accused me and his father of being controlling. Everything was our fault, according to him. The therapist promised things would get better. But he is not a teenager anymore, and his issues continue. It's very hard.

THREE FAMILIES: THREE STORIES

"This just isn't happening. It's a nightmare and I'm going to wake up and be so relieved," said Maura, when she learned that her twenty-three-year-old son was arrested for cocaine distribution. Maura and her son lived in an upscale suburban neighborhood, miles away from where drugs entered the city. "I could not conceive that Tim could get caught up in a drug web. So I thought this just had to be some terrible mistake." Sadly for both of them, it was not.

In another case, Jack remembers learning that Sarah, his thirty-five-year-old daughter, had left her husband and three kids to run off with a stranger. The man was fourteen years younger than Sarah, and had started as Sarah's drug connection. Their relationship was propelled by her supply of money, his access to drugs, and their shared dependency on heroin. "That just came out of nowhere," says Jack. "As soon as I figured out what she did, I knew then that her life, my grandchildren's lives, and my life would be forever different."

Barry was a college junior when he returned home a few semesters short of graduation. A growing depression and social anxiety disorder made it impossible for him to continue. Taking solace in his old bedroom, weeks turned into months. Even with treatment, his progress was minimal. Many times the university reached out to Barry and asked him to re-enroll. Barry had a great incentive to return because his scholarship depended on it, but he missed one deadline after another. Barry's parents were initially very supportive, but soon his father's patience waned. Every interaction with his son became vitriolic. His father said, "How can you let this scholarship go? How can you do this to me and your mother?" The less Barry responded, the more biting were his father's words: "Whatever is going on with you—well let me tell you, it's enough. Just get it together. You hold your end of the bargain. Stop acting so selfishly."

Emotional Reaction: Denial

At first, Jack could not speak with anyone about the episode with his daughter. His wife was exasperated with his emotional inaccessibility. She pleaded with him to talk about it. Jack was stunned and seemed to believe that if he did not discuss it, then it did not happen. Jack's wife complained, "I am at war with my daughter's actions and my husband's denial."

When a body responds to a threat, the "fight or flight" mechanism kicks in. Hormones and neurotransmitters surge, the heart beats stronger, blood pumps furiously into the muscles, and the body is ready to fight back. It's hard to identify what happens in the brain immediately before this chemical cascade, but there is a brief moment of disbelief before we fully size up a threatening situation. The physiological changes prompt the psychological reaction of denial. Denial should be understood as a temporary safe harbor that protects you from reacting too quickly. It exists because your mind and body are not ready to process the enormity of the blow. For better or worse, shock and denial are short-lived and the full force of the problems will hit you soon.

Emotional Reaction: Guilt and Self-Blame

The evidence against Tim regarding his cocaine arrest was insurmountable and soon he had no other choice but to come clean. Maura was angry at him for his arrest and for being so unrepentant.

After her initial shock, Maura felt compelled to take inventory of what she had done wrong. With her therapist acting as her sounding board, Maura said, "I wonder if we gave Tim too much? I did not think I was spoiling him, but we never made him work, we sent him to summer camp, and he has been to Europe twice. Maybe he turned to drugs because nothing else was a challenge?" At her next visit to the therapist, Maura had developed another theory for how she could have been a more effective parent. "I should not have let him go to college in the big city. This is where he met the other guys in the drug ring. I should have demanded that he go to a small rural school. I just wanted him to be close by."

When told by her therapist that drugs pervade every strata and every college, Maura could not listen; she had already moved on to yet more self-incrimination. "We should have restricted him from video games. I think Tim was inspired by them." Again Maura's therapist tried to reassure her, saying, "Most parents make some mistakes raising their children, but you probably erred no more than your friends whose children are thriving.

Tim's decisions were his choices, not yours." It took a skilled therapist to convince Maura that her child's path to self-destruction would not have been altered even by the most perfect parents.

Emotional Reaction: Anger

Anger often spills over when parents stew in the aftermath of their adult child's problem behavior. Like denial and like guilt, anger is a natural emotional response to your child's predicament. It's understandable. At times, your child needs to hear your anger. If he steals something or hurts someone, then he needs to hear your condemnation. At other times, as with Barry, your child's problems are due to a medical or psychiatric condition over which he has little control. Angry words only intensify the problems.

GIVING UP ON THE FEAR AND THE DRAMA

Sometimes my daughter (age twenty-three) is as sweet as can be and then at other times, she's the meanest person imaginable. One moment she might say that I'm her very best friend and then she will get frustrated for some reason and announce that she hates my guts and wishes that I were dead. I have tried to emotionally disconnect from her, which makes me sad and causes lots of guilt. But I'm tired of all the ups and downs. I'm tired of the drama.

Emotional Reaction: Anxiety and Depressed Feelings

To be a parent is to know anxiety. Anxiety begins in the delivery room even before you complete the ten fingers and ten toes checklist. It continues when children start school and crescendos the weekend before you learn whether he has made the varsity team or as you wait to see if she was chosen for a coveted job. But these agonies are transient; parents recover quickly from these moments, certain that they will be replaced by other mundane concerns.

In contrast, the demands of parenting a troubled adult child are unrelenting. Chronic stress can develop into heightened anxiety and clinical depression for a parent. Jack discussed his response to his daughter's abandonment of her children: "I alternated between panic and fear. I could not imagine how we could rebound from this. I continued to play out the likely scenarios. My grandchildren would go with their father. He would never let us see them. My wife would never forgive our daughter. I would stay awake all night alone with my negative thoughts." Individuals who have a past history of anxiety and depression are more vulnerable to new episodes when their children sweep in and disrupt their world.

If you become depressed or develop severe anxiety, it becomes a challenge to emotionally support your family. You may need treatment yourself to help fortify you, and we strongly suggest that you seek the help of a mental health therapist in such a case. Be open to the therapist's suggestions,

---

STRESS-BUSTING EXERCISE:
ASK YOURSELF WHAT YOU DID RIGHT

Why did this happen to my child? You might think it's because you're a single parent or because money was tight when your child was growing up or because you worked too much—there are endless ways to blame yourself. Here's an exercise to combat those distortions. Get a paper and pen or create a new computer file. Then record the positive aspects of your relationship with your adult child. Instead of agonizing over what you did wrong, consider what you did right.

Push yourself and come up with a minimum of three examples. They can be simple: You bathed and clothed and comforted him when he had the flu at age six. When he got older and started to get into trouble, you stood by him, when everyone else gave up. You did your best in good and bad times. You got him hospitalized when he was suicidal. You gave him life and probably have saved his life.

Don't hesitate to list other achievements and grade yourself generously. Then file your notes away so you can easily retrieve them. Whenever your negative thoughts return, pull out the document and read it aloud. Internalize it. You're not all bad and you're not all good. No one is. Welcome to the gray space where most parents live.

---

which may include counseling or medications. Much of this book discusses the psychiatric issues that explain your troubled child's behavior. Chapter 9 offers solid recommendations about how to approach your own mental health needs.

BEHAVIORAL REACTIONS

Along with your emotional reactions to your adult child's problem behavior, you may also experience behavioral changes, including irritability, social isolation, and alterations in your appetite and sleep patterns. You may also notice an increase in your alcohol intake. Many of these behaviors can be helped with the input of your physician.

Irritability

In times of turmoil, you might find yourself lashing out. Janet relates that when she learned that her son had received his third DUI, she was mad at the world and made no pretense at hiding her rage. She recalls screaming at a convenience store clerk who didn't give her the correct change. (To her embarrassment and the clerk's irritation, the change *was* correct.) Irritability can intrude into the lives of normally even-tempered people. When you are struggling to make sense of your adult child's seemingly inexplicable behavior, it's hard to completely contain your feelings of frustration. Sometimes the least deserving people—other family members, coworkers, and even the check-out lady—become the target of an imprudent outpouring.

WHEN ADULT CHILDREN ARE VIOLENT

My son is thirty-six and he scares me. He was arrested for punching his girlfriend when she was pregnant with their first child, and he was ordered by the court to take anger management classes. He took them. But I'm guessing that these classes did not really solve his problem, because the anger is still there, in full force.

Self-Isolation

If you feel wounded by your adult child's behavior, you may start avoiding your old friends and even steer clear of your extended family members, turning down invitations to family reunions, birthday parties, and holiday events.

In a support group for parents of troubled children, Erica spoke of her daughter Amy's uncontrolled manic behavior. When Erica was with her close friends and family, she did not know how much information to share about Amy. On one hand, they were sympathetic, but on the other hand, Erica wanted to protect Amy from their judgments.

Erica's husband, Peter, also felt such conflict. "Don't share our problems," he implored Erica. "They will not understand what you're going through and they will get tired of hearing about your problems." Peter believed that most friends and family would offer phantom support; they would say the right things, but on some level, they would assume that Erica and Peter were flawed parents and were now reaping what they had sowed. But when Erica avoided the topic of her daughter when she was with her friends, her conversations quickly started to feel forced and false, and she felt alienated and alone.

Every family draws their boundaries differently, but to avoid self-isolation, it's necessary to cultivate relationships with those who truly understand your feelings and vulnerabilities. Support groups of parents with troubled adult children (like the one in which Erica later shared her feelings) can help. You certainly can't avoid family and close friends forever, but you should remember to apply some ground rules. For example, if you talk openly about your child one day and later, in a fit of self-reliance, entirely avoid the subject, your friends will be unsure of what they can ask you. At the same time, try to avoid over-talking about your child's issues. This may be very hard to do, since this subject dominates your thoughts. Friendship means sharing, but it should not be a one-sided monologue of woes.

I'll Have One More

You may find yourself turning to alcohol more frequently when you are overwhelmed. This response is understandable, but alcohol has an insidious way of making things worse. It may reduce anxiety initially, although over time most people have to consume a larger quantity of alcohol to get the same relief. There are so many reasons to minimize and to manage your use of alcohol. Alcohol is difficult for your liver to metabolize and it can damage your gastrointestinal tract. It is a central nervous system depressant, and when used in high volume over a sustained time period, it will depress your mood. Alcohol distorts judgment and impairs memory. It is the essence of all addictive substances: appealing and helpful in the moment, but a full-blown disaster over the long run. Moderation is the key.

In tough times, compare your current alcohol consumption to the amount you drank *before* you got caught up in your adult child's problems. Take notice if your routine of a drink before dinner starts to include two drinks after dinner. Inform your doctor if you can't reverse this trend. She will help you find resources to get some control.

Changes in Your Appetite and Weight

Weight management is a constant struggle for many Americans; over-wrought parents are as vulnerable as any in this daily battle. Karen fought obesity throughout her adult life, and she frequently subjected herself to restrictive diets. Several years ago, she underwent lap-band surgery and lost nearly 120 pounds. But when Karen's adult son was accused and ulti-mately convicted of sexually abusing a teenager, she lost all control over her eating routines. During the two years of the legal proceedings, she gained back most of her weight. In light of her emotional distress, the thought of waging another weight loss campaign overwhelmed her. "This fight is over," she told her doctor. "The surgery was my trump card and I already played that hand. I don't have the strength to start again."

Another patient, Alan, struggled for years with intestinal malabsorp-tion, a medical condition that left him chronically underweight. In order to maintain his health, he labored to consume thousands of calories daily. But these efforts were interrupted when Alan's twenty-five-year-old daugh-ter abruptly left home, persuaded by her online boyfriend to move from Michigan to Salt Lake City. She disappeared for eighteen months until a private investigator found her dancing in a topless bar outside Reno. She agreed to come back to her father's home, but by this time Alan had lost twenty pounds and his internist ordered a feeding tube to replenish his weight. Even after she returned home, Alan had no greater control over her. His daughter quickly resumed prostituting to support her oxycodone dependence. In his weakened condition, Alan couldn't intervene and he found this sense of futility impossible to accept. His daughter's behavior continued to consume him, both figuratively and literally.

Both Karen and Alan experienced a significant and unplanned change in their weight as a result of their ongoing heartache. Weight gain or loss is evidence that an individual has lost control of established routines. Weight changes might also signal the onset of depression or another mood disorder and in such cases, your doctor should be contacted.

SHE'S GLAD HER SON CAN'T HAVE CHILDREN

Mario is thirty-five years old, and he is unable to have children. I could not handle the worry if I had a grandchild that he or his wife was raising. There are drugs and alcohol all over their house. Mario is a long way from getting clean and sober. Thank God there are no children to worry about.

Tears Are Flowing

There are few disappointments greater than witnessing your adult child fail. Each parent, whether they admit it or not, harbors hopes for their children. Hopes can be modest, as with, "I want my child to be healthy and gainfully employed," or more ambitious, such as "I hope my child makes the big leagues . . . I want him to go to Wharton just as I did."

Most parents adjust their expectations as they distill an honest appraisal of their children's capabilities. At some point, parents realize that some of their previous dreams were idealized. In general, however, disappointment comes in degrees. While it's unsettling to realize that the ten-year-old child whom you hoped would follow your championship example is actually pretty clumsy, recognizing that your thirty-five-year-old is someone who will lie and manipulate others is far more painful.

Each separate realization may come with a behavioral reaction. In a Families Anonymous meeting, Jose's mother shared her devastation on learning that her son had become HIV-positive from his intravenous drug use. "I have not been able to stop crying for weeks. I can barely function at work because I can't stop crying. No one wants their accountant blubbering over tax returns." A few days of crying lie within the normal range for most people, but if it continues for weeks or months and interferes with your daily life, then treatment is appropriate. Hint: Antidepressant

---

STRESS-BUSTING EXERCISE:
TREAT YOURSELF AS YOU TREAT OTHERS

One stress-busting technique is to imagine a social conversation with other people who struggle with their adult children. Consider Amanda who tells you about Max, her twenty-seven-year-old son who is morbidly obese and not working. She says, "I feel that if his father and I had stayed together or at least not have had such a nasty divorce, then things would have turned out better for him." Do you agree with Amanda? Do you tell her that, yes, she did a *really* bad job and Max's problems directly spring from her parenting? Of course you don't. You might silently ask yourself what role Max has in his own poor performance, but it probably would not occur to you that Amanda's divorce was solely responsible for her son's fate.

Now turn your attention to your neighbor Sam. His son Bill's cocaine addiction cost Bill his job and two years in prison. Bill's wife divorced him and moved a thousand miles away with Sam's grandkids. Sam said, "I'm not sure what I did wrong with Bill, but it must have been something."

Do you agree with Sam? No, as with Amanda, nothing you know about his parenting could have forced his adult child to make such bad life choices. You remember Sam as an excellent father who took Bill to karate clubs and drum lessons. You encourage your neighbor to think about better times, and tell him with great sincerity that he did the best that he could as a parent.

Now, take the next step. You *are* Amanda. You are Sam. Why not cut yourself the same break as did the friendly and caring outsider? Every time you start to berate yourself for your inadequacies, reframe the situation and think how you would advise someone in the same situation.

medications can control tearfulness within a few days. See chapter 7 for a full discussion about psychiatric medications.

BLAMING GENES

Jenny and Jeffrey have been married for thirty years and both see the same psychiatrist for different problems. Jenny has long been stable on ADHD medication and Jeffrey has done well on an antidepressant. In their separate meetings, both lament the plight of their twenty-nine-year-old son Adam, who never completed his education, held down a job, nor lived independently. And although they rarely talk about it to each other, each finds the other one culpable for Adam's situation.

Jeffrey, perhaps half kidding, says that he has little respect for Jenny's family and sees Adam as the natural extension of generational mediocrity. For her part, Jenny has developed a complex genealogical theory that traces Adam's faults to her husband's gene pool. She reminds their doctor that on Jeffrey's side of the family, "At least four people went to jail for something. Jeffrey's father was an alcoholic and his brother never worked a day in his life." This shared frustration has led Jenny and Jeffrey into constant accusations.

Should science find one day that a specific behavior is linked to specific genes, then their arguments might seem more valid. That day has not yet come and even if it does, you still cannot control which genes you pass on to your children. Does this mean that parents are not responsible for their child's outcome? No. We absolve parents not because all the decisions they made for their children were perfect, but because perfect decisions would not have ensured their children's well-being. We dismiss Jenny and Jeffrey's carping because genetics alone do not dictate how children turn out. Multiple factors—genetic, environmental, and sociological—account for how a child matures into adulthood. The following chapters try to make sense out of this complicated calculus.

STRESS-BUSTING EXERCISE: THOUGHT BLOCKING

Sometimes recurring thoughts can become problematic and can impede psychological healing, and in such cases, a simple technique that cognitive-behavioral therapists call thought blocking may help. With this technique, you can run interference with recurring problematic thoughts. For example, let's say you keep thinking, "It must be my fault that Sharon is an alcoholic." Then each time you start to "hear" in your mind the beginning "It must be my fault . . ." immediately say to yourself, "No!"

After a while, the negative thoughts will occur much less frequently, and when they *do* intrude, you can learn to challenge them by replacing them with other positive thoughts, such as "I did my best and it's not my fault." (Cognitive-behavioral therapy, a very helpful approach for parents of adult children with serious issues, is also described in detail in chapter 9.)

KEY POINTS IN THIS CHAPTER

- Distressed parents experience anger, disbelief, guilt, and self-blame.
- Common behavioral reactions of a distressed parent may include self-isolation, yelling and screaming, and blaming others.
- Distressed parents may gain or lose weight and may drink too much alcohol.
- Blaming your spouse or partner for the genes brought to the relationship is not productive.

The next chapter covers the problems that are inherent in living in the same house with your adult child who may be violent, mentally ill, or abusing drugs or alcohol. Even if your adult child does not live with you, you may find helpful suggestions in chapter 3, and we recommend that you at least scan it.

IF YOUR ADULT CHILD LIVES WITH YOU

At least my husband gets to go to his office. I work from home, and my son with atten-
tion deficit lives with us. I watch him playing video games and drinking beer all day
long. If I ask him to do anything around the house, he can get really angry with me.
So far he has not hurt any of us, but he has punched many holes in the drywall. He
also threatens me. I am worried that one day if he gets too upset, he will lose control
and become aggressive. He seems right on the edge.

All parents hope that their children will excel in sports or demonstrate some artistic talent or academic or entrepreneurial skill that will position them for success. Many times, parents find this satisfaction in some of their children—how sweet it is to witness your child flourish. Unfortunately, no family receives a guarantee that all their children will succeed. In many ways, life is a lottery and even Bill Gates's parents could have had another child who came up well short of the mark. We must strive to be loving parents to them on both graduation day and the day they are released from a psychiatric hospital or a correctional facility.

On the most basic level, the rhythms of any mature household will be disrupted when your home includes a troubled adult child. Most parents are not ready for the onslaught of unpredictable behavior and tirades of abusive language, and the situation can deteriorate quickly. Possessions may not be safe, and art and jewelry that you bought years ago can be pawned in a snap. Violent behavior can also be directed against beloved family pets. The difficulties are compounded if your innocent grandchildren move in.

Parents may disagree about whether it is wise to allow their adult child to return home, but the urgency of the moment often leaves no choice. Furthering the uncertainty, parents may not know how long their children will remain or whether the children can pay their share (or any) of expenses. There may be insufficient time to calculate the needs of grandchildren. As a result, parents often feel powerless and unprepared to meet these sweeping demands.

There are steps that can be taken to improve your home situation, and this chapter focuses on the best methods to communicate your expectations and establish proper boundaries with your troubled adult child. The need for adult children to return to their parents' home for any lengthy time usually signals some fundamental difficulty with maintaining their independence. Often mental health and substance use disorders are at the core of this struggle. For these reasons, families of adult children with issues must learn to negotiate around the American mental health system. This chapter concludes by examining this structure and offering tips on how to communicate most effectively with your child's mental health team.

WHO RETURNS HOME?

Children who are forced to return to the parental home usually fall into three major categories. The first group includes young adults in transition. They might move home after college and before they find their first job. They might also return home to continue their education, to live cheaply while they plan their next venture (for example, a move to another city) or to save money for a house down payment. These reunifications can be rocky—too many adults living under the same small roof can be trying. Nevertheless, these are passages of life and most families survive them just fine.

The other two groups comprise more troubled individuals. First, a large number of these young adults have substance use disorders (SUDs) with alcohol and/or drug issues or they have antisocial personality disorder (ASPD). While SUD and ASPD are both considered mental health conditions, experts are divided as to whether these individuals are willfully self-destructive or if their behavior is better explained by an underlying brain illness. Some of the pessimism about SUD and ASPD among mental health professionals is that the conditions, particularly ASPD, do not respond well to available treatments. These conditions often co-occur with other, very treatable psychiatric conditions. For instance, people with ASPD or SUDs may have ADHD, bipolar disorder, or depression.

Psychiatrists spend a significant amount of time distinguishing socio-pathic actions from a bad action caused by another psychiatric illness. Major mental illnesses such as chronic paranoid schizophrenia or bipolar disorder are undeniably brain-based illnesses. Unlike with SUD and ASPD, psychiatric medications clearly help with these major mental illnesses. (See chapter 7 for a fuller discussion of these conditions.)

WHEN YOUR CHILD COMES HOME

It is devastating to realize that your child has become the person whom most of us fear: the one who has abused a child, misused drugs, commit-ted crimes, or participated in one antisocial activity after another. They often end up in the criminal justice system. These adults experience many life transitions: between jobs or between relationships or between jail sen-tences. During this flux, families feel forced to provide their adult child with a place to stay while attempting to help him plot a path forward.

PRACTICAL ADVICE

No two scenarios are exactly alike and no two families respond to these complicated challenges in the same way. Still, it is wise to develop some general guidelines so that expectations are known and the lines of author-ity are clearly marked. While parents are at the top of the power structure, the velvet glove usually works better than the iron fist. The following sec-tion offers practical guidelines for a healthy coexistence with your adult child:

- Stating to your adult child what the family needs instead of stating "what's best" for the child
- Concentrating on one problem at a time
- Picking your battles

Effect Changes by Stating What the Family Needs

Many parents make the mistake of telling their adult children how they should behave. "Take your medication, don't spend all your time online, stop provoking others with your insulting language," are refrains that are echoed in many households. The underlying implication is that it would be in the adult child's best interests to modify his behavior in a manner that is acceptable to his parents. However, this approach often leads to a belligerent reaction, such as "Don't tell me what I want. I don't need anyone to tell me what to do." Instead, it is far more productive to persuade her by stating clearly what the family needs.

Here are two examples. Most of the rest of the world operates during the day and between 9:00 a.m. and 5:00 p.m. If your child has any hope of getting a job or otherwise integrating into the mainstream of society, you know that she will need to avoid staying up late at night and then sleeping until noon. Yet the argument that your prickly adult child needs to maintain a regular sleep schedule will likely be rejected. So take another approach.

Instead, package your advice in the context of what's good for the family rather than what's best for the individual. Keep it simple and tell him that one person preparing food, listening to loud music, or engaging in other activities in the middle of the night keeps other family members awake, and it would be best for everyone in the family for him to get into a regular schedule. It's hard to argue with that.

Similarly, while parents understand the doctor's advice that psychiatric medicines need to be taken as ordered, your comments about the benefits of taking the pills regularly may be completely lost on a self-defeating adult. Reframe this issue in more concrete terms.

Ask your adult child to take his medications on schedule for the family's sake. You may say, "We notice that when you take the medications you are less anxious and irritable and we fight less as a family." This approach allows your child to make a concession to you and the family, one that he does not perceive as personally controlling.

Adult children with serious issues can be oppositional and proud. They may argue with you not because they disagree with you but rather for

THOUSANDS OF DOLLARS
WITH NOTHING TO SHOW FOR IT

We spent thousands and thousands of dollars trying to help our son, who is an addict. We even bought him land with a trailer. He was mad that we wanted to charge him a small rent, and so he tore up the trailer. When he moved out, even the land was a mess. He always returns back home, but every time, it is a disaster.

the emotional stimulation that comes with conflict. They may object to the notion that other people, especially their parents, could know better than they do what is good for them. Still, as a parent, you cannot allow yourself to be intimidated or have your voice silenced. You simply have to communicate your point artfully. The chart on page 41 lists common conversations and suggests some effective methods to restructure your responses so that you can avoid having the same arguments repeatedly.

Concentrate on One Problem at a Time

Most adult children described in this book have multiple issues. Their problems can range from financial issues to housing to basic health concerns, and it can be hard to know just where to start. In some situations they may have lost the capacity for basic judgment.

"I feel that she needs so much," stated the mother of a twenty-four-year-old cocaine abuser. "She eats terribly, her skin has broken out, and she has gained a lot of weight. She refuses to get up at a reasonable time in the morning and she is not showering or putting on clean clothes."

In general, it is best to use a gradual approach to these problems. Sweeping change is unlikely to occur overnight, so instead, concentrate on one problem with your child at a time.

Instead of unrealistic pronouncements that from now on, your daughter will be required to rise by 8:00 a.m., adopt a vegan diet, and consult with a dermatologist for her skin care, choose the behavior that bothers you the most and insist that you need *that* behavior to change. For example, the body odor and dirtiness may bother you the most, so make this

Often Said/Better Said

Often Said	Better Said
Pick up your room because you need to live in a clean space.	Please don't eat in your room and get rid of any food that's already there, because we don't want to get ants and other bugs in our house.
You can't bring weapons in here because you might harm yourself.	We don't allow anyone in the family to have guns or other dangerous weapons in our house because they're too dangerous for family members.
You shouldn't bring your bad friends in the house because they might use drugs here.	Please don't bring people in the house who have known criminal records or who are violent. They could harm someone in our family.
Don't stare at family members because it makes you look weird.	Please don't stare at family members because it really makes them feel uncomfortable.
Don't lose your temper and bust holes in the wall or kick in your door. It's better for you if you're calmer.	If you bust holes in the wall or kick in the door, you scare other family members and then we also have to hire someone to repair the damage. Please try to find ways to calm yourself before you damage property.
That stupid dog is your responsibility and not mine! Take care of him or I will really take care of him!	We don't like it when your dog has accidents on the carpet or somewhere else in the house. The dog will have to leave in the next few days if he has any more accidents.
You are filthy and you stink! It's disgusting.	You don't smell nice and it really bothers us. Please take a bath or a shower.
Stop yelling because it makes you look like a maniac.	Please stop yelling because it is very upsetting to other family members. Let's try to discuss the problem calmly, either now or later.
Take your medication because you need it.	Please take your anxiety medication because your agitation and irritability is really upsetting everyone, even the dog.
You shouldn't eat late at night because it's bad for you.	Please don't prepare food late at night because when you do that, you wake sleeping people up and it's upsetting.

the priority. She must take a bath or a shower on a regular basis. Even the most compromised person can handle one behavior change. And when she does comply, enjoy the moment and congratulate her for her success. Later, you can move on to the next most pressing issue.

Pick Your Battles

The above approach does yield results, but you can't move too fast. Said Dan, the father of an adopted son with ASPD as well as a severe learning disorder, "My son can't stay organized, and he makes a mess wherever he goes. This is a problem because my wife and I crave order in our home. We made this point many times to our son, particularly before we left for a short trip. When we returned we were so happy that the living room looked good. He was really delighted to hear the compliment. Then I looked at his bedroom in the basement. What a mess! Junk everywhere. It looked like a scene from one of those hoarding programs on TV."

This is the time to bite your tongue if you have to before you blurt out your first response. Instead, regroup and think about the situation. Your son is understandably proud that the living room looks great, and he clearly made a dedicated effort to make it that way. It is more important that the shared family space is tidy compared to his bedroom. Positive reinforcement such as praise is the most effective way of changing another person's behavior and on some level, even troubled adult children want to please their parents.

So pick your battles. Praise him for the living room. Later, explain calmly that next time you would like him to tackle the mess in his bedroom. If you explode too early, then you defeat the benefit of the progress that was made.

BEWARE OF THESE BEHAVIORS

By using some of the above strategies, parents of problem adult children can help to restructure the balance of power within their homes. Parents of adult children with ASPD regularly confront terrible behaviors. In the next few pages, we explore the dangers that these adult children may bring into your home. These behaviors may happen repeatedly, and it is important to recognize their seriousness and plan what you will do when your adult child:

- Purposefully damages your home and property
- Invites people to your home that you think are dangerous
- Brings weapons or other items that you consider dangerous into your home
- Brings illegal drugs into your home
- Makes verbal or physical threats against you or other members of your household

Damage to Your Home or Property

Adults with ADHD may be severely impulsive and may damage property. They may become frustrated very quickly and they cannot direct their anger effectively. They commonly slam doors, punch the walls, or damage the furniture. Unlike people with pure ASPD, they feel remorse after the outburst. They typically recover rapidly and move on as quickly as they had become angered. Typically their family members are considerably less emotionally resilient—and they also tire of plastering over the drywall. If your adult child is diagnosed with ADHD, share with his doctor how he reacts when he is frustrated. Changes in medications can help.

More ominous are adult children who use property damage or the threat of weapons as a means to frighten or control their family members. Family members may see evidence of BB gun damage in the house or they may notice an adult child's fondness for setting fires within the home. These individuals are likely to have antisocial personalities and they have little remorse for their actions. In addition, this property damage can be a warning sign of further violence. In these cases, you may need to distance yourself from your adult child, particularly if the violence seems to be escalating or you sense that you are in danger. (Read the discussion in chapter 12 about when you need distance between you and your child.)

MY SON USES PEOPLE

My son has always attracted a lot of attention. He is striking to look at and since he was little, people would go out of their way for him. I noticed that he never returned the affection. People are interchangeable to him and he quickly sees how he can use them. He is just cruel.

He sleeps with men who are vulnerable, either with some sort of emotional problem or who have issues about how they look. He has conned them out of vast quantities of money before he disappears out of their lives. He has also conned me out of large sums of money.

Inviting Dangerous People into the Home

Jayne registered her displeasure at a Family Anonymous meeting. "My husband and I served in the Navy and we have seen a lot. Two years ago our son moved home. Most of his friends scare me. A couple of them drive loud trucks and have terrible white supremacist tattoos. My neighbors are really uncomfortable with all the activity."

Just as when your son or daughter was sixteen, it is still your home and you can decide who enters your property and who must go. Your adult child probably won't like it, but if he wants to keep these friends, he can visit them somewhere else. Follow your gut. If your inner voice is screaming an alarm to you, then something is wrong. Heed it. Don't let people in your home who scare you.

Weapons

Never allow your troubled adult child to bring a gun, large knife, bow and arrow, or any other weapon or disturbing item into your home. It doesn't matter whether you believe in the right to bear arms or are a life member of the National Rifle Association. That is irrelevant in the case of a troubled adult who is mentally ill or a substance abuser. Also, if your child has been convicted of a felony in the past, he loses the legal right to possess a gun.

If you observe a weapon in your house, tell your adult child that either it goes or he goes, and if he refuses to remove the weapon, make sure he leaves the house with the weapon. If he later returns, tell him to empty his bags before he enters the house or at the entry to your home to make sure he is minus any weapons. You have the right to ban guns in your own home. It is of course your right to keep them yourself, but the wisdom of having deadly force near an unpredictable adult child is debatable. Weapons can be used for protection, but they can also be used against you. If you do keep weapons, store them safely.

Illegal Drugs or Misused Prescription Drugs

Never let your adult child bring in illegal drugs (such as marijuana, cocaine, or methamphetamine) or abused prescription painkillers (such as hydrocone, oxycodone, Oxycontin, or Xanax). Of course, your child may bring in and hide such drugs without your knowledge. But if you do see such drugs or you smell the sweet odor of marijuana in the house, then tell your son that the drugs must go or he must go.

This warning is given not only for your own protection, but also for the protection of others in the home. Every year there are reports of small children who have died from ingesting discarded medications. It is also true that some street drugs can lead to increased aggression or violence, particularly cocaine or methamphetamine. In addition, if the police should suspect illegal drug possession in your home, they can enter your house with a search warrant—sometimes in the dead of night for the surprise factor.

If you are aware that drug use continues, then follow through with your threat. Calmly advise your adult son or daughter that they have twenty-four hours to be out of your home. If they miss the deadline, then put their possessions out on the front lawn. Call the police, and tell them you suspect your child of illegal drug activity. This is not easy to do at all! But protect yourself and your other family members.

Verbal or Physical Threats

Troubled adult children often were troubled youth, and thus, their parents are not strangers to verbal and physical threats. If this happens when they are adults, it is essential to try to ratchet down the situation. Raising your voice or arguing back will further escalate the tension. Attempting to refute the logic of your child's arguments will only worsen the situation. Instead, speak in a controlled voice and a lower than normal tone. Remember, your child's outbursts are not rational discourses. There are no debate points that will be scored here. It is irrelevant whether you are "right" and the other person is clearly wrong. When you are threatened, no matter the age of your child, the most important issue is defusing the current situation and staying safe.

Avoid staring at your angry adult child and never touch her when she is enraged. If she requests something and you can do it, then do so, even if the request seems silly or stupid to you. Offering food or a soda is a great way of turning down the heat.

It is important to manage the crisis, but when your adult child threatens you, it means that he can no longer live in your home because you are not safe. Violence perpetrated by adult children can and does happen and no parents can be expected to live in fear. Parents also have the option of seeking a restraining order. This edict establishes a physical radius within which your child may not enter. If he violates this space, the police may remove your adult child from your home. Sometimes a few days in jail can resolve the crisis.

You are not a failed parent if you take this action, and you let your adult child go to jail; you are acting prudently. Most mentally ill people are not violent, but do not assume that your adult child would never harm you. Adult children have injured or even killed their parents and family while in the throes of rage, psychosis, or a reality that is impaired by drugs and alcohol.

For many parents, obtaining a restraining order is a difficult line to cross. Leora recalled the dark moment when she petitioned the court. "I can't believe that I did it but I am so glad my counselor urged me to take action," she said. Leora's son had repeatedly threatened both her and her husband.

Leora said, "I saw that when my husband gets angry, my son becomes ballistic. I had to protect all of us or someone was going to get hurt." For

Leora's son, the restraining order led to a psychiatric hospitalization and treatment with antipsychotic medications. Leora had accurately assessed her son's situation. She also knew that the threat to her own safety was far too great for her to manage alone. Restraining orders can always be lifted, but the failure to act in the face of danger can result in an irreversible physical injury for the victim and a lengthy prison sentence for the perpetrator.

CONSIDERING MANIPULATIVE BEHAVIORS

Even if your adult child has been diagnosed with a serious psychiatric disorder, it is still possible that she may use manipulative behavior to convince you to do whatever she desires, be it giving her money or allowing menacing people into your house. Realize that a psychiatric disorder is an explanation and not an excuse. For example, if your son says that he is too tired to vacuum for you, then he should be too tired to go fishing with his pals. This is true whether your son is eight or twenty-eight. Other examples of manipulative behavior are provided in the chart on page 48 to help you distinguish a real problem from an excuse.

IF YOUR CHILD EXHIBITS PSYCHOTIC BEHAVIORS

Some bad behavior can be calculated, but individuals experiencing psychosis have little direct control over their actions. Parents struggle with the best approach to their children's auditory hallucinations or persecutory delusions. Auditory hallucinations are internal voices that command the individual to behave strangely. Delusions are fixed false beliefs that often revolve around the theme that others, including you, have ill intentions against them.

Parents of psychotic children quickly learn that their psychotic behavior cannot be readily reasoned with, and that it is nearly impossible to talk anyone out of their symptoms. To your child, the symptoms feel profoundly real. She really *hears* those voices in her head and she actually *sees* those images before her, and she has no doubt that the threat against her,

**Examples of Manipulative Behavior
versus Likely Nonmanipulative Behavior**

Action You Request	Response of Adult Child	Later Actions	Is This Manipulative Behavior?
Please take out the trash.	I can't do it because I'm too tired.	Person is invited to a party or to do something he likes, and he agrees.	Yes, this is manipulative. If he's too tired for doing simple tasks, then he should be too tired to do fun things.
Please take your medication.	I don't like it because of the side effects.	Person refuses to take medication.	Possibly manipulative. If the person is concerned about side effects, then he should consult with his prescribing doctor.
Please stop yelling at me.	I'm yelling at you because you caused all my problems!	Person continues to yell.	Probably manipulative. Person may believe that you caused all his problems. Or he may know that you're a self-blamer and be using this to hurt you.
Please come to dinner.	I'm too upset.	Someone calls and invites her to dinner and she accepts.	Yes, this is manipulative.

sometimes perceived as posed by her family, is accurate. You can, however, mitigate the negative and harmful effects to yourself and to your other family members.

This section covers the following recommendations:

- Try to put doubt in their minds over delusions and hallucinations and offer reality checks.

- If your child becomes violent, make sure you are between him and the door.

- Change your behavior to cope with paranoia.

- Don't accept your adult child's self-injuries, such as cutting, without taking action. Cutting is a sign that psychiatric treatment is urgently needed.

Offer Reality Checks

Although you can't talk a psychotic person out of his delusions and hallucinations, you can tell him that you don't believe what he believes and you don't see what he sees. Assure him that you know that these sensory experiences are very real to him—but it's not your experience. At best, you can put some doubt in his mind about what is going on. Conversely, if you actively try to talk him out of the tricks his mind is playing on him, this is a battle you will not win.

Mentally ill people are not the only individuals who may hallucinate and exhibit psychotic symptoms. In some circumstances, drugs and alcohol can cause psychotic behavior.

Don't Let Him Get Between You and the Door

Don't imagine or assume that your adult child would never harm you, particularly if he or she is behaving in a very threatening or aggressive manner. Consider possible escape routes if the anger seems to be escalating. If you can't get out the front door, what about other avenues of escape? Consider them all and leave if you have to. If you can't leave because your adult child is much faster than you are and blocks your exits, then call 911 for help.

Change Your Behavior to Cope with Paranoia

If your adult child seems to believe that you or others are acting against her (paranoid delusions), take the following actions.

- Do not look a person in the eyes who is exhibiting active paranoia. This can be viewed as a direct threat. This can be hard advice to follow when it's your own child. But do it anyway.

- Avoid using pronouns such as "I" or "you" in your conversation, and instead use vaguer ones such as "they" or "we." This is less threatening language when dealing with a paranoid person.

- When the person is confrontational, try to stand next to the individual rather than looking her straight in the face. Assume body language that implies that you're together in this thing.

Don't Accept Some Behaviors, Such as Cutting

A person who self-injures, as with cutting, may be trying to find release from their internal emotional pain. But you cannot allow cutting to continue: Your adult child could cut herself more severely than she intends, and the cuts could become infected. But above all, the internal emotional turmoil revealed by cutting means that the person urgently needs help from a mental health professional.

WORKING WITH MENTAL HEALTH PROFESSIONALS

If your child has mental health issues and he is treated privately, a psychiatrist is usually the primary clinician. Under ideal circumstances, the psychiatrist works closely with a therapist. However, in the United States today, most individuals with chronic mental illness are cared for in the public mental health sector.

Most community mental health centers (they go by different names in different states) provide care using multidisciplinary treatment teams. These teams are usually led by a psychiatrist and include a combination of nurses, psychologists, and pharmacists. Many times case managers are assigned. These professionals are often social workers or licensed professional counselors. The psychiatrist is ultimately responsible and often adds her expertise with diagnosis and medication management. Psychiatric nurse practitioners also manage medications and they offer other therapeutic services as well. Psychologists often perform psychotherapy, as do clinical social workers and licensed professional counselors. The treatment team divides up responsibilities for their clients. Some team members are experts on housing, and others are focused on helping their clients integrate into the employment world. Social workers often act as the liaison between the patient and his family.

The teams may work together for years, communicate at regular intervals, and after a few years of experience, become unfazed by the challenges they face daily. Most teams humbly recognize that the time they spend with your child is limited and to truly understand how their patient is functioning, they must get information from family members who are living under the same roof. Collaborative working relationships are ideal, but it does not always work that smoothly.

At times, families become frustrated with the care that their adult child is receiving. In private practice, the psychiatrist and the therapist may practice in different offices and this limits their ability to communicate freely. The left hand may not know what the right hand is doing. This poor coordination is less likely to happen in a community mental health center, but it does occur.

Patrick's family spoke poorly of his treatment team. "In our case, the team kept changing. We had trouble knowing who was making decisions or why they were made." Ryan's parents complained, "The doctor never told us anything. Our son was causing chaos in our home and we could not communicate with the psychiatrist. It felt like we were the enemy. We felt that the mental health professionals were not interested in what we had to say."

Improving the Relationship Between Parents and Their Child's Doctors

Technically, there is no relationship between you and your adult child's mental health professionals unless your child specifically grants you the right to obtain information from them. However, even if your child refuses to grant such permission, you can still provide information to the treatment team and hope that it will be useful.

Here are some key points to keep in mind.

1. Realize that information cannot be shared freely without a medical release. The Health Insurance Portability and Accountability Act (HIPAA, pronounced as "hip-ah"), a federal act, forbids medical professionals from disclosing private medical information even to other family members unless the ill person has granted such permission.

    As a result, think ahead. It is always smart to have these releases signed well before a crisis arises, having obtained them at a calmer time. You might require such releases from your child as a precondition for allowing her to live with you or assisting her in any other way. Once a release has been signed, a free flow of exchange can occur between you and the treatment team.

2. If you are unable to secure this release from your adult child, do not despair. There is nothing forbidding parents from informing the treatment team about their child. The team may not be able to respond to you, but your information is vital and will be helpful in the overall scheme.

3. Tell the treatment team if your child is not taking his medications. Many times behavioral disturbances may be treated by medication changes. For example, tell the team if your child is "cheeking" his medication (holding the medication inside the cheek so that it can be spit out later), or if you notice that the bottle of medicine is still full weeks after it was dispensed by the pharmacist. Treatment teams often depend on family members who live with the patient for this information.

4. If possible, find out why your adult child is refusing to take her psychiatric medication. Medication noncompliance can be due to a patient's overt decision not to take their medication. Other times, noncompliance can be due to a problem with disorganization or a faulty memory. In these situations, the treatment team can help the family develop simple behavioral techniques to increase the likelihood that the medications will be taken on schedule.

    For example, placing medication in a weekly plastic box divided Monday through Sunday prompts the patient to take the medication daily. At the end of the week, there is also a clear record of how many doses have been missed. It is helpful to place the medication box next to the patient's toothbrush, as most adults will brush every morning and when they do, they'll see the pill container and be prompted to take their morning medications.

5. Inform the treatment team if and when your child demonstrates serious mood swings, violent outbursts, or new behaviors, such

as abusing drugs or alcohol. Many times the team can intervene and change the medications or make psychotherapeutic interventions. Safety is a primary goal and the team has experience with local laws and customs regarding an involuntary commitment to psychiatric facilities. The local police or sheriff can be called upon in emergencies, and these potential situations are best discussed with the treatment team before you encounter a crisis.

CONSIDERING MANDATED ACTIONS AND TREATMENT

Sometimes decisive interventions are needed. Individuals with mental illness who present a threat to themselves via suicide or a violent threat to others may be committed for involuntary psychiatric hospitalization. Generally this process starts in an emergency room when a physician determines that the patient poses an immediate threat. The doctor then certifies the findings to the probate court and the court decides if the hospitalization is legally justified. Most states do not allow involuntary hospitalization for individuals with active substance use disorders or Alzheimer's disease or other forms of dementia.

In recent years, state laws have expanded the definition of which persons require treatment. This movement has encouraged outpatient psychiatric care. In forty-four states and the District of Columbia, the court can order mentally ill adults to take their psychiatric medication. This is known as outpatient or assisted outpatient treatment. (This option is not available in Connecticut, Maryland, Massachusetts, Nevada, New Mexico, and Tennessee.) To find out what the laws are in your state, go to this website offered by the Treatment Advocacy Center: treatmentadvocacycenter.org/solution/assisted-outpatient-treatment-laws or search online for your own state laws.

Many commitment laws are cumbersome and many families find it difficult to access appropriate care in a crisis. For this reason, many states have adopted patient advocate laws. These reforms allow individuals with a history of mental health treatment to designate a friend or family member to act on their behalf while they are mentally incapacitated. For example, in the event that an individual with bipolar disorder becomes manic or psychotic, their designee can decide on the need for treatment rather than waiting for a probate court to act. The decision to designate a family member or trusted friend should be done when the patient is well. The necessary paperwork can be facilitated by the local community mental health board.

Some people believe that these laws are violations of an individual's civil rights, despite the fact that they have been upheld by the courts. But the severely mentally ill person often has an equally severe lack of insight into their own illness and their symptoms, which usually can only be resolved by treatment, including psychiatric treatment, therapy, and medications.

The conversations between a patient and his therapist are usually confidential unless a threat is made against a third party. In these circumstances, mental health professionals have a duty to warn others. Although these laws are designed to protect innocent parties, the therapeutic alliance is often irreparably broken when therapists report concerns about their patient to the police. The National Conference of the State Legislature's website details state laws: ncsl.org/issues-research/health/mental-health-professionals-duty-to-warn.aspx.

KEY POINTS IN THIS CHAPTER

- Practical advice includes picking your battles with your child, stating what the family needs, and solving one problem at a time.

- Some behaviors should not be tolerated, such as your child bringing weapons into the home, making verbal threats, or committing physical abuse.

- If your child is psychotic, you need to change your own behavior, such as making sure you can leave the home during a violent episode if necessary.

- Talk to your child's physician and try to seek a release from your child to do so. If you can't obtain a release, you can still share important information, such as that your child has stopped taking his medication.

Child abuse and neglect is covered in the next chapter.

PART TWO

TYPES OF PROBL[EMS]
BEHAVIOR AND [WHAT]
YOU CAN AND CAN'T DO

Part Two covers specific problems that adult children may exhibit, such as substance abuse issues, mental illness, child abuse, criminal behavior, and suicidal behavior, with one chapter for each topic.

CHAPTER 4

BAD PARENTING

Sandy, fifty-three, knew her daughter Carly, twenty-two, lived on the edge. Through-out her adolescence Carly had smoked marijuana and had made bad choices in friends. When she was twenty, Carly started to use cocaine and alcohol. Sandy knew this was dangerous behavior not only for Carly but also for her three-year-old son, Domingo. That Carly refused to listen to her mother's concerns at all left Sandy feel-ing helpless and desperate. But Sandy felt like she could not turn her own child in to social services for being a bad parent, could she? After all, she had little proof that Domingo was in danger so far and he seemed fine.

Everything changed the day that Carly passed out from her substance abuse, and Domingo walked out the front door and into a busy street, narrowly missing get-ting hit by a bus. The bus driver called the police and social services was contacted. Domingo was placed in foster care. After caseworkers decided that his grandmother Sandy was competent and willing to care for Domingo, he was then transferred into her home. Social services and the family court also developed a case plan for Carly to follow. If she wanted to get Domingo back, she had to complete a drug rehabilita-tion program and seek follow-up substance abuse and psychiatric care. She was also ordered to take parenting classes and get a job.

Sandy and Carly were lucky that Domingo was not injured. Other children are not so lucky, and they are harmed and sometimes die because of parental neglect or outright abuse.

When adults are impaired by mental illness, substance abuse, or other issues, they are more prone to neglect or physically harm their children. Be aware that it may happen, and be prepared to take action if it does. Your adult child may not be taking his psychiatric medications, or he may be abusing substances—or sometimes both. You may need to become the temporary or permanent caregiver to your grandchildren.

THREE ESSENTIALS TO HELP ABUSIVE PARENTS RECOVER

Sometimes parents who have lost custody of their children say that they want the children back, but they may be unwilling and/or unable to take the actions needed to be parents again. There are three essential factors in resuming custody of their children, including acknowledgment of the problem, the ability to resolve the problem, and the means to resolve it. If all three are not present, then the problems that led to the abuse or neglect will not be resolved.

Acknowledgment of the Problem

If a parent is told by social services or others that they have a specific problem, whether it is drug abuse, an abusive boyfriend or girlfriend, or another problem, if the parent refuses to agree or even acknowledge that there is a problem, then the issue will remain unresolved. For example, if a live-in boyfriend beat a child, caseworkers will likely say that this man must move out. Yet some mothers will resist, saying that they need him or that it's not "fair" that he should have to move out. In another example, if a parent has a drug problem, such as the abuse of prescription opioids such as hydrocodone or oxycodone, but he insists that he has complete control of the issue and refuses treatment, this is another failure to acknowledge the problem. This failure to acknowledge a problem is a key issue among people accused of abuse and neglect, even when there is clear-cut evidence of the drug problem.

Ability to Solve the Problem

In order to resolve a serious problem, a person needs to be *able* to solve the problem. For example, if the adult child is developmentally delayed, she may need extra help to care for her child because on her own, she cannot provide appropriate care. If she is ill with a serious disease, she may also need help. The inability to solve the problem may be intellectual, mental, or physical.

Having the Means to Solve the Problem

The abusive or neglectful parent also needs the means to solve the problem. For example, if she needs a job but does not have a car, and bus transportation is not available, then she may consider it impossible to get the required job. However, in most cases, caseworkers will work valiantly to provide the means needed to solve problems preventing the parent from being a good parent.

SOME BASICS ON ABUSE AND NEGLECT IN THE UNITED STATES

According to child maltreatment statistics provided by the US Department of Health and Human Services, in 2011 676,569 children nationwide were abused or neglected. As in previous years, children ages three years and younger suffered the greatest risk for all forms of maltreatment except sexual abuse.

Some states provided data on whether the child had a caregiver who was an alcohol abuser or a drug abuser, calling this a risk factor for abuse or neglect. The federal researchers found that in about 19 percent of the cases of maltreated children, there was a caregiver abusing drugs. They also found that in about 10 percent of the cases of maltreated children, there was a caregiver abusing alcohol. Thus, children living with caregivers who are substance abusers, particularly drug abusers, have an elevated risk for suffering from abuse or neglect.

In considering children who died from child abuse or neglect in 2011, the researchers found that the greatest percentage of child deaths (about 17 percent) occurred in families with domestic violence issues, followed by those with drug abuse issues (13 percent) and then alcohol abuse issues (6 percent).

One of the most important studies on child abuse was published in 2012 by L. Jones and colleagues. They concluded that physically disabled children were nearly four times more likely to be treated violently than were nondisabled children. In addition, the children with intellectual or mental disabilities had a nearly five-fold greater risk of suffering from sexual violence than did the children without these disabilities.

Consequences of Child Abuse to the Adult Child

Excuses or explanations such as mental illness or substance abuse generally do not resonate with judges or juries when children are abused and neglected. As a result, and particularly if the abuse or neglect is severe or is fatal to the child, both the parent and his spouse or partner may end up in prison.

Even if the perpetrator avoids being sent to jail or prison, she likely will be placed on the state child abuse registry. Abusers will suffer the humiliation of being on the registry, but more importantly employers will not hire them, under the assumption that anyone who harmed a child once may well repeat their behavior with other children. Service jobs that involve children or the elderly are out of reach to those on the child abuse registry. This drastically limits employment options and serves to increase the dependency that these adult children have on their parents.

WHEN CHILDREN ARE ABANDONED OR NEGLECTED

As difficult as it is to believe, nearly every day in the United States, someone leaves a baby or small child unattended. Sometimes they leave a child in a hot car in the summertime, tragically causing the child's dehydration and death. Sometimes parents leave an infant in the care of other small children while the parent goes out. The parent may be unable to pay for child care and may rationalize that they need their money for other purposes. There are so many ways that small children can get into trouble when left alone that it's impossible to list them all here.

Think about if you have ever spent time childproofing a home when a toddler is living with you or even visiting your home. Vigilant parents cover the electrical outlets, block lower cabinets where toxic cleaners are stored, and lock away all knives so curious children do not find them. In contrast, parents who neglect their children typically do not foresee life's potential dangers, and as a result, they are much less capable of protecting their children from potential risks, let alone from the adult's own problematic behaviors, such as using drugs or alcohol to blot out their own emotional pain or mental illness symptoms.

When Children Are Abandoned

Abandonment is one of the worst kinds of child neglect. Veteran abuse experts tell haunting stories about child abandonment. Children have been left unattended during their parents' work shift and sometimes for much longer periods. Newspapers occasionally report terrible cases when a parent has forgotten that the infant is in the back seat of the car, only to find the child injured or dead hours later.

Sometimes these cases are tragic mistakes, but other times a parent's neglect can be traced back to mental illness or substance abuse. Psychosis, driven either by schizophrenia or by drug abuse, can become so intense that the individual loses all perspective of time. Their instinct for self-care disintegrates, and they become incapable of tending to their children's needs. They may assume that someone else will step in or somehow believe that the kids will be just fine. This kind of magical thinking helps the parent to justify the abandonment.

When Children Are Neglected

In addition to abandonment, children are neglected when their parents fail to meet the child's basic needs of food, shelter, and medical care. Physicians can tell if a child is an appropriate height and weight for his age—*if* the parent brings the child for regular medical checkups.

Sometimes, often for unknown reasons, some parents have singled out one child to deny him basics such as food and water, and shockingly emaciated children have been discovered by child welfare workers after someone has alerted them. In such cases, all the children in the family are removed, including the healthy ones, because the remaining children are

---

SHE WISHES HER DAUGHTER WOULD COMMIT A CRIME

I wish my daughter would commit a crime so I could pursue custody of her two-year-old daughter. My daughter has been diagnosed with depression and an anxiety disorder and her life is in constant chaos. The constant worry about my granddaughter drives me crazy. But since my daughter is not a raging drug addict or abusing her child, the state won't do anything.

---

believed to be at risk for such neglect in the future. For example, if the ill child is removed from the home, the disturbed parents who harmed him may identify and single out another child as someone to be harmed or neglected.

"Medical neglect" may also occur, when sick children are not taken to the doctor for an evaluation. Every child should have a pediatrician or family doctor and every parent should be familiar with the local hospital emergency room in case it is needed. In virtually all states, children have protected access to medical services. All hospitals must care for the emergency needs of children. Parents with no money or with limited financial resources can apply for Medicaid for their children. The application process may become a barrier. Immigrants who are in the country illegally worry about declaring themselves to government authorities. Other parents may forego Medicaid because it requires filling out forms and providing basic documentation. Some are unable to organize themselves to follow basic procedures.

ABUSED LITTLE BOY

My grandson came to live with me when he was three, about two years ago, and the state placed him with me because of his mother's abuse and neglect. This little boy's life had been very chaotic with my daughter. When he was with her, he'd go to bed after 2:00 a.m. and then sleep most of the day. I put him on a normal schedule.

When he first arrived, this sweet little boy was very fearful about making mistakes and he constantly apologized to me. He once told me to not ever make his mother mad because it was not good at all to make her mad. He didn't give me any more details and I was afraid to hear them anyway.

I have a restraining order against my daughter now because she came into my house once with men carrying guns and she was verbally and physically abusive to me, right in front of her little boy. She also threatened that she was going to take him away and drive across state lines until she was caught. She hasn't seen the child for months now because she refuses to accept visits with him that are supervised by a caseworker. But the child still loves her.

HER NEGLECT BEGAN AT BIRTH

When Emma was born weighing only two pounds, she was immediately transferred to the neonatal intensive care unit (NICU). Emma's premature birth left her with many conditions that jeopardized her life. Her parents, Nicole and Kyle, decreed that no one could visit Emma unless they gave express permission—which they withheld from everyone. Kyle's parents objected but were told by the hospital that, by state law, the wishes of the birth parents superseded the grandparents' pleas. Kyle's parents knew that Nicole had severe ADHD, but since Nicole's mother died, Nicole had refused to take appropriate medications that controlled her impulsivity.

In recent years, Nicole had used marijuana and cocaine, and to ensure a ready supply of drugs, she made bad friends and bad choices. Emma was conceived after Nicole had let her birth control prescription lapse. Nicole and Kyle visited Emma only rarely during her three-month stay in the NICU. The hospital staff knew that parents of other premature babies visited daily and they feared that Nicole and Kyle were not responsible to care for their child. The NICU social worker reported the case to child welfare services. Kyle's parents were alerted at this point and became immediately involved. They later deduced that Emma's parents had banned them from the hospital because Kyle feared they would discover that he and Nicole rarely visited and that they would withhold money as a punishment. Nicole did not want to be forced into treatment.

Unsafe Environments

There are many types of unsafe environments, and it doesn't always take a trained eye to spot it. Many public health officials assert that children exposed to cigarette smoke are at risk for upper respiratory illnesses. However, this risk is dwarfed by the threat from illegal drugs. For example, the introduction of crack cocaine has devastated families in American cities. Young women have experimented with crack and developed addictions so consuming that they endangered their children. Over the last decade, many states also have been flooded with the scourge of methamphetamine. Methamphetamine is a vile addiction on many levels, including the fact that it is often manufactured at home. Children can be exposed to toxic fumes and there have been many reports of fiery explosions engulfing family homes where meth is cooked.

Emma's neglect continued after she was discharged from the hospital. After starting strong, Nicole began to miss her scheduled outpatient appointments, and the doctors again contacted child protective services. Eventually, the medical neglect led to Emma's removal from her birth parents and into a placement with Kyle's parents. A year after Emma's birth, Nicole had not entered treatment and Kyle and Nicole had left the state. Emma continued to stay with her grandparents and soon became physically healthy. Last year she entered kindergarten and she is the earliest reader in her class. Kyle eventually returned to his hometown and found employment. He visits Emma regularly at his parents' home, but has not assumed or sought custody. He does pay his parents a portion of his income to support his daughter.

Sadly, however, Emma's mother, Nicole did not recover. She remained drug-dependent and continued to refuse treatment. She has brief periods of stability but has danced in strip clubs and has become an escort to support herself and her habit.

Emma's grandmother told me, "It was a difficult decision to make to raise Emma ourselves, but when we made the decision, we did it with our heart and soul. We think Emma and Kyle are better for it. Our world revolves around Emma and though we expected our retirement to be a little different, it is hard to imagine it being more gratifying."

PHYSICAL ABUSE

Stories of overt physical abuse of a child are the most chilling. Abuse can take the form of slapping a child for misbehavior or dunking the child's head repeatedly into the toilet—essentially waterboarding the child for not potty training fast enough. Abusive parents sometimes force small children to eat entire bars of soap for "talking back, a potentially fatal action."

In a high profile murder case of a small child, it was alleged that the mother used chloroform to sedate her child so that she could go out and party. The child did not survive and her body was later located. There are occasional cases of mentally ill parents interpreting command hallucinations to beat the demons out of their children. The use of illegal drugs often increases aggressiveness. In one horrific case, a parent injured his son, age four, after using the hallucinogenic drug phencyclidine (PCP). The boy later said, "Daddy ate my eye."

If You Think Something Is Wrong, But You're Not Sure

Sometimes you can't quite put your finger on it, but you feel like your adult child could be endangering her children. But you need more than a bad feeling to report to social services staff about potential abuse or neglect. Most state social service agencies are very underfunded and understaffed, and often it is difficult for protective service workers to keep up with needed investigations of abuse or neglect allegations. It is also true that more than half of all the reports to child protective services in the United States are eventually determined to be unfounded, which may mean that nothing happened *or* it could also mean that there was insufficient evidence to determine that abuse occurred and that the state agency should act.

To gain an idea of what's really going on, it is wise to visit the home where the children live. If you see squalid conditions that appear dangerously unhealthy or you witness a child's injury or the child being hurt, assume the abuse continues and report these conditions to the social services department. (See Appendix C for a state-by-state listing of child abuse hotlines.)

When you are with the children under your care, whether you are at your home or you're in your adult child's home, be sure to take a long, hard look. If you can answer "yes" to any of the following questions, then abuse or neglect concerns arise.

- Are the children covered with bruises?
- Do the children have broken bones, and do these fractures recur?
- Are there an inordinate number of bug bites all over the child's body?
- Are the children alert and healthy?
- Are they clean, with no ground-in dirt under the fingernails?
- Do the children seem very fearful of their parents or someone else who lives in the home?

Also, take a look at the home environment where the children live, and if you can answer "yes" to any of these issues, there is likely a problem, especially if the children are infants or toddlers.

- If there are pets, do the animals seem healthy and well fed? Check for whether the pets look sickly, dirty, or too thin. People who mistreat pets may also mistreat their children.

- Are the children dressed inappropriately? A toddler who is playing outside in the snow in sandals and a sleeveless shirt and shorts is clearly not dressed right for the weather.

- Is there a smell of urine about the house?

- Can you see fecal material inside the house, and no one seems to notice or care?

- Are there dangerous objects that are present and accessible to the children, such as guns or knives?

- Are cigarettes and butts left lying about and accessible to small children? (Small children can consume cigarettes or cigarette butts, which are harmful and may be fatal.)

- Is alcohol left about and easily accessible to the children?

- Is there a distinct odor in the house that may be from the use of drugs? If you inquire what "that smell is," do you receive laughter or no response at all?

When to Call Social Services

If you are worried that your grandchildren are in danger, but for some reason, you are not willing to call the abuse hotline, be sure to check up on the children at least every few days. Don't just call them—go to the apartment or home where they live, so you can see how they look. You may find they are alone and hungry and scared. You may find that they are fine.

In some unstable situations, you cannot assume that if the children are fine on Monday, then they will still be fine on Friday, especially if your adult child's behavior is making all of your alarm bells go off. Check the children again on Friday. And if you see anything that causes concern at that time, then call the child abuse hotline. If your adult child is already working with a caseworker, call that person. You're not "ratting out" your child. You are working to save your grandchildren.

WHEN GRANDPARENTS BECOME PARENTS

Some readers will be caring for their grandchildren or may soon be caring for them because of an issue with their adult child. Sometimes the process takes a long time, but when a child finally enters the foster care system the state tries to place him with a close relative. Grandparents, aunts and uncles, or siblings of the abusive parent are frequently approached to assume this responsibility. In these desperate situations, middle-aged or older adults find themselves parenting, sometimes for the first time. It is hard to imagine a greater challenge.

If you become your young relative's caregiver or legal guardian, take total control. The child is your responsibility now: Do not let a situation develop that gives you pause. For example, if your adult child is allowed to visit her own child, do not allow unsupervised visits until you are comfortable that the past abusive behavior will not be repeated. Demand that the parent receive treatment and let him know that he must prove to you that he is compliant with treatment. Insist that a current release of information is signed so that you can have open communication with your adult child's treatment team (see chapter 3). With the assistance of child social services, you can and should control the level of exposure that the young child has to his parent, and it should all be done on your terms.

Some Basic Do's and Don'ts for Visitations with the Child
Here are some basic do's and don'ts to consider if your adult child is allowed to visit your grandchild.

1. Do keep the child at home during visits or meet the parent at a public place, such as a park. Do not let the parent take the child anywhere alone, not for a walk down the street and certainly not anywhere in a car. The parent may decide this is an opportunity

to take the child back. Think how frightened and confused the child will be, and especially after the police are forced to track down both your child and your grandchild.

2. Do listen in on ongoing conversations between the child and the parent to make sure that nothing is said which is frightening or threatening to the child and that no false promises are made (such as, "You're coming home again really soon!"). Yes, it's okay to eavesdrop when you're trying to protect a child.

3. In the same vein, don't let the child talk on the phone to a parent unless the speakerphone is on and you can readily hear both sides of the conversation. A parent who feels angry or threatened may say very disturbing things to a child, and if so, you need to know about this.

4. Don't accept rude behavior or foul language from your adult child during visits to children. If such behavior occurs after one warning, tell the adult the visit is over.

5. Keep in mind the person whom you are protecting: the child. You may feel sorry for your adult child and empathize with the distress of not having the child at home, but the key person, the child, is under your care and should be your priority. Remember, it is up to social services and the court whether the child is returned to the parent. It is also up to the parent: If the parent fails to do what social services has said must be done in order for the child to be returned, then this failure is not your fault or your problem.

KEY POINTS IN THIS CHAPTER

- To recover, abusive and neglectful parents need to acknowledge the problem and have the ability and the means to solve it.

- Evidence of child abuse may include severe bruising, fractures (especially recurrent breaks), or extreme fear of the parent.

- Evidence of child neglect may include an extreme number of bug bites, failure to take sick children to the doctor (medical neglect), and inappropriate clothing (such as thin summer clothes when it is snowy and cold outside).

- It's very hard to call a state abuse hotline when it's your adult child who is the abuser, but you need to do so to protect the abused or neglected children.

The next chapter covers the distressing situation of when your adult child commits crimes.

CHAPTER 5

CRIMINAL BEHAVIOR

Jenny opened the door to the impatient police officer. He needed to speak to her daughter about a complaint that she shoplifted from the local Nordstrom's. Jenny was shocked. Sure, Mandy, age twenty, had some issues, but she did not need to steal. She worked full-time and the family was generous to her. Jenny told the officer that Mandy wasn't home at the time but she was due back in about an hour. He said he'd be back.

When Mandy returned home, Jenny was relieved that she adamantly denied the allegation. But, sure enough, the officer returned and showed them a picture of Mandy leaving the store with expensive boots. She could not supply a receipt. Resigned, Mandy left quietly with the arresting officer.

WHY PEOPLE COMMIT CRIMES

Criminal acts are motivated by many factors, greed and cold calculation chief among them. People commit crimes because they think they will get away with them. Others lack a moral compass.

In many cases, psychiatric conditions lead to criminal behavior. For example, some individuals with obsessive-compulsive disorder (OCD) feel a compulsion to shoplift, perhaps to complete a collection or to add to a random horde. Others, who have ADHD, are attracted to the thrill of shoplifting and cannot resist the excitement of getting caught. Those with drug dependencies steal because they are addicted and need funds to sustain their purchases.

Whatever the explanation for this behavior, many parents are forced into the criminal justice system to help defend their adult child. There are few things more perplexing for a parent than to watch a child go astray. If his problems are longstanding, you likely did whatever you could to set him on a firm footing. And if nothing worked, you probably blamed yourself. If his criminal problems started later in life, you might indict your child, his peers, or his living situation. But feelings of guilt are there, and parents always try to answer the nagging question: What could I have done better?

This chapter is intended to help parents cope with these trying times. We include a basic primer that helps you navigate through the criminal justice labyrinth. We also offer tips about how to respond when your child gets into trouble. The premise of *When Your Adult Child Breaks Your Heart* is that psychiatric issues are often at the core of aberrant behavior. Individuals with mental health problems are more likely to be involved in the criminal justice system, whether as perpetrators of violence or as victims of crime. If you find yourself in this difficult circumstance, we encourage you to ally with your child's attorney so that you can advocate for your child's treatment needs. Hopefully a greater understanding of the relationship between mental illness and criminality will allow you to guide your family through tough terrain.

A PRIMER ON THE CRIMINAL JUSTICE SYSTEM

Parents of troubled adult children often have time to learn about the criminal justice system. Many of their children have had contact with the police and courts for years. The earliest contact might have been in adolescence for using alcohol or dealing marijuana. Minors convicted of larceny or assaults likely have served time in juvenile detention, a system that may appear cozy compared to the harsh punishment doled out to adults.

Occasionally the first contact your child has with the system occurs in adulthood. These parents have little familiarity with law enforcement or the courts other than a long-ago traffic ticket or what they have seen on *Law and Order.* Cop shows teach us that people who are accused of crimes are entitled to certain rights such as the right to an attorney if they cannot afford one and the right to remain silent. But aside from those glimpses offered by television dramas, the criminal justice system is largely a mystery, and most families are intimidated by the criminal process.

Some Basics
Adult crimes are divided into two categories: misdemeanors and felonies. Prosecuting attorneys assess the details of an alleged crime and determine

at what level to press charges. Misdemeanors are lesser crimes and they may include petty theft, minor vandalism, and driving while intoxicated. The court often offers probation to first-time offenders and they are spared jail time if they complete the terms of probation. Probation may last a year or two and might also include community service, regular check-ins with a probation officer, and periodic drug testing. The court has little patience for probation violators and repeat misdemeanors, and sentences up to a year duration in the county jail are common.

Felonies are serious crimes, such as burglary and assault, and violent crimes like rape and murder. Felonies are punished severely, although repeated misdemeanors such as multiple driving under the influence violations may be elevated to felony status. Convicted felons are sent to the harsh environment of the state prison, housed alongside violent offenders serving long terms.

Bail is money that is paid in order to allow a defendant to leave jail until his trial date. Whether bail is granted and the amount of the bail is determined by a judge, based on state laws.

Bail is handled differently in different states. In many states, bail is paid through a bondsman, an individual licensed by the state to act as an intermediary between the person paying the bail and the court. Some states allow a percentage of bail to be paid through a bondsman, while other jurisdictions require the entire amount be paid upfront to the court. Bail is granted contingent on the defendant not leaving the state and showing up on his court date. If he fails to appear on the appointed date and at the appointed time, the bail is forfeited, and a warrant will be issued for his arrest.

When It's the First Time (As Far As You Know)

The first time that your adult child is charged with a crime is probably not the first time that he has actually committed a crime. While this might be a statistical fact, most parents of adult children initially contest their child's involvement. Many convince themselves that the allegations must be a terrible error, a case of mistaken identity or a gross miscarriage of justice. Calls are often made to retain the best defense attorney. Families hear arguments that an established private attorney will have greater sway over the court's decisions than less experienced public defenders. Whom to hire is one of the first of many decisions families are forced to make as their child enter the criminal justice system.

SOME TIPS

Here are some basic tips for parents of adult children who have been accused of crimes. Learn from the mistakes other parents have made.

- Do not assume your child is innocent and don't listen to lies.
- Do not rush to hire expensive attorneys.
- Do not rush to bail your child out of jail.
- Do always insist that your child receive mental health treatment.

Do Not Assume Your Child Is Innocent and Don't Listen to Lies

Unfortunately with bad behavior, past is often prologue. Unless a significant change occurs in your adult child's life, such as a mental health intervention, the risk of your child repeating negative behavior is quite high. Sure, he may well be innocent of the crimes of which he's accused. And our legal system assumes innocence until the defendant is found guilty by the courts. But when you learn that your child has been charged with a crime, it's natural to assume that the cops have arrested the wrong man. This assumption may lead you in the wrong direction.

Consider the very real possibility that your child *may* not be innocent. Parents know their children well, and usually there are hints of inappropriate behavior before the authorities become involved. Many crimes are an extension of established patterns of behavior. If your daughter is accused of theft, rethink her past before rushing to her defense. Has she ever stolen any items from you? It is typical for people who resort to stealing from strangers to have first victimized their family.

If your child is accused of possessing illegal drugs, consider if there were warning signs. Has his behavior changed of late? Has he been fired from a job for tardiness or for not following rules? If your daughter is accused of distributing illegal drugs, consider whether she used drugs in the past and now may be so addicted that she is forced to deal drugs in order to maintain a fix. Similarly, an adult arrested for violent behavior usually has demonstrated a past history of poor self-control. In their honest moments, parents, cognizant of their child's past behavior, may be shocked that their adult child has been caught, but not that surprised that he has been accused.

For other parents, it may be difficult to maintain an objective stance when your child swears up and down that she is innocent. Mandy, the twenty-year-old described earlier, harangued to her mother that she was unfairly accused of shoplifting, yet she relented the moment after she was confronted by an incriminating security camera image. Others will continue to insist on their innocence despite overwhelming evidence.

Lying may be a recurrent issue for your child. Of course people tell white lies all the time. But many parents of troubled adult children realize that their child easily lies about everything. Pathological liars lie so often that they cannot keep track of all their deceptions. Lying starts early in life and develops into a reflex after the child's early realization that it can deflect blame. Later in life, they recognize that getting away with the lie is so psychologically reinforcing that it becomes a habit, particularly if they find themselves in frequent trouble.

Do Not Rush to Hire Expensive Attorneys

Everyone who is accused of a crime needs an attorney, and families often struggle over who should represent their child before the court. If your child has little money or convertible assets, then she is entitled to a no-cost public defender. Public defenders are notoriously overworked and relatively inexperienced.

Private attorneys usually require a large retainer, often ranging from $4,000 to $25,000 or more, depending on the complexity of the case. In general, private criminal attorneys are more experienced than public defenders and have deeper support personnel.

Choosing the private option for a legal defense may make sense for a family with resources. If the charges against your child are unfounded or the consequences are so significant that you want the finest representation, then it may be worth retaining private counsel. Still, there is no guarantee that clients of a private attorney will have a better outcome than if they were represented by public defenders.

Several years ago, I testified about the psychiatric condition of a young pediatrician who was accused of fondling one of his adolescent patients. The doctor's defense attorney, who had received a large retainer, had an excellent reputation that had been recently bolstered by the local media's coverage of his successful defense of two police officers accused of murder. But the lawyer was ill prepared to take on another complicated case so soon. He prepared no defense exhibits, offered weak cross-examinations, and was unfamiliar with the details of the case. The pediatrician was convicted and sent to jail for eleven years. I cannot say for certain that he was innocent, but it was clear that he received a weak defense. The defendant learned a tough lesson; you don't always get what you paid for.

This story may be an exception and parents may still opt for private counsel. The pediatrician's father later told me that he was comfortable with his decision. "My son may be locked up for a while, but I needed to know that I did all I could to help him. It would kill me if he was convicted or had a longer sentence because I did not pay for the best lawyer." It becomes harder to maintain this enthusiasm for paying for expensive counsel if your child is a repeat offender.

One point is very clear. The most important factor to ensure a good defense is to communicate with your child's attorney. Help her obtain all the facts and encourage your child to communicate with her in a productive manner. An attorney, private or public, will do a better job if she trusts you and your adult child.

Keep in mind that your child is not automatically entitled to your money or your indiscriminate financial support. Public defenders can also secure a fair outcome. As a parent, you are naturally worried about your child's future, but you have every right to protect your own security as well.

Do Not Rush to Bail Your Child out of Jail

There are certain issues that families encounter unexpectedly and have to decide in haste. It's worth considering certain scenarios ahead of time.

What if your family dog suddenly becomes ill and needs surgery? Are you willing to pay thousands for emergency surgery that may extend his life for a few months? How would you respond to a call from a relative in need of a kidney donation, someone with whom you have little emotional connection? All sides of these ethical debates can be argued and good people inevitably will reach separate and valid conclusions. Similar dynamics face the parents of troubled adult children as they grapple with the immediate decisions regarding bail for their imprisoned child.

The judge sets the amount of bail for individuals charged with a crime but not yet convicted. In the short run, the payment of bail releases the accused from jail and gives him time to work on his defense. It is also a powerful incentive for him to show up for trial, lest the bail be forfeited. Families of those accused the first time are usually eager to extract their child from jail and work furiously to raise enough money to make the required amount.

Our Internet survey reveals that in retrospect, some families question their initial zealous reaction. Grace's son Todd was arrested for possession of narcotics with the intention to distribute. No one in her family had been arrested before, and the first time Grace had been inside a jail was the day she visited Todd. She was appalled by jail conditions and the coldness of the corrections officers even to families. Bail was set for $50,000 and the family was required to come up with $5,000.

In the panic of the moment, Grace reached out to a family friend who was a veteran police officer. He advised Grace to "Let him cool off in there for a few days." He predicted that after a week in detention, the judge would lower the stiff bail. The brief stay behind bars would give Todd time to think about the bleak implications of a longer incarceration.

Grace dismissed her friend's advice and gathered the money. Within twenty-four hours of his arrest, Todd was released from the county jail. He returned home barely impacted by the experience. Todd did appear for his trial, but he acted arrogantly, a posture that may have contributed to his conviction and harsh jail sentence.

Todd's years behind bars were miserable, and his toughness at trial did not translate into fitness for jail. Looking back, Grace wonders if she had not bailed Todd out so quickly, if he might have acted differently before the judge. Her hasty rescue was a lost opportunity for him to learn a timely lesson.

Do Always Insist That Your Child Receive Mental Health Treatment

If you suspect that your child has a mental illness, be sure his criminal attorney is made aware. Work to obtain a diagnosis and treatment for your child before his trial date. If the crime resulted from mental illness, for example, assaulting a police officer during the manic phase of bipolar disorder, the court will take this into account. The presence of mental illness certainly will factor into how his case is prosecuted and might be a factor in obtaining a more humane sentence from the judge.

Be wary of a lawyer who dismisses the mental health aspect of your child's case or who contends that the court's knowledge of his psychiatric condition would work against him. This is a sign of a lawyer trying to take a shortcut away from a complete defense.

VIOLENT CRIMINAL BEHAVIOR, MENTAL DISORDERS, AND SUBSTANCE ABUSE

Some research indicates that individuals with mental disorders, especially those with bipolar disorder or schizophrenia, have an increased risk for violent behavior. The risk for violence escalates further if a seriously mentally ill patient abuses street drugs. Other research shows that mentally ill people are more likely to be victimized by others and are susceptible to domestic violence and homicide. There is new evidence that the treatment of certain mental illnesses, specifically ADHD, decreases the risks for more criminal activity.

Research on Violent Criminal Behavior

Researchers have demonstrated that the risk for violence increases when a person has a mental illness, and the risk increases markedly when the individual has both a mental illness and a substance use disorder. In a study reported in the *Archives of General Psychiatry* in 2010 of adults with bipolar disorder, 21 percent of those with bipolar disorder and substance abuse had committed violent crimes, compared to only 3 percent of the non-bipolar controls who were violent and only 5 percent of the subjects with only bipolar disorder and no substance abuse. Clearly, the combination of bipolar disorder and substance abuse is a risky one. Mental health professionals should consider both bipolar disorder and substance abuse issues when they evaluate violent behaviors.

Another study drew on data from the National Epidemiologic Survey on Alcohol and Related Conditions (NESARC). The researchers evaluated nearly 35,000 subjects and closely examined patients with schizophrenia and a mood disorder. Among subjects without serious disorders, the prevalence of violence in the past year was less than 1 percent. When the person had a serious psychiatric disorder (as occurred in 2,531 cases) but no substance abuse disorder, the prevalence of violence was about 3 percent. In the population with both a serious mental disorder *and* a substance use disorder, the rate of exhibiting violence was about 10 percent, more than three times greater than the group with the psychiatric disorder alone.

The researchers also examined the relationship between criminality, anxiety disorders, and personality disorders. Only about 2 percent of individuals with these conditions exhibited violence over a one-year period. However, when anxiety disorders and personality disorders were combined with substance use, the rate of violence more than tripled.

The message for parents of troubled adult children is clear. Mental illness complicates one's life, but adding the substance abuse dimension substantially elevates the risk for violence.

Mentally Ill People Have a Higher Rate of Being Victimized

Individuals with mental illnesses may become criminals, but they are also often the victims of violence. A British study performed by Christina Hart and colleagues explored the relative risk of victimization among the mentally ill. Using data from the National Child Development Study, their rate of criminal victimization in the past year was 18.2 percent, compared to 14.5 percent for the non–mentally ill. In addition, 3.5 percent of the mentally ill had suffered from violent crime in the past year, more than double the rate of violence sustained by those without mental illness. The authors said, "A prior history of mental disorder was found to be a robust predictor of criminal and violent victimisation."

Trevillion and colleagues looked more carefully at domestic violence. They analyzed the results of studies of individuals with depressive disorders, anxiety disorders, and post-traumatic stress disorder (PTSD). Individuals with these conditions were at greater risk of suffering from domestic violence than individuals without them. For example, women with depressive disorders had nearly three times the risk for domestic violence as women who were not depressed. Women with anxiety disorders were four times more likely to be victimized at the hands of their partner than non-anxious women. A past history of trauma increased a woman's vulnerability to further trauma. Women with PTSD were seven times more likely to suffer domestic abuse than the rest of the population.

The mentally ill are also at greater risk for being killed. In 2013, Swedish researchers found that mentally ill people were about five times more likely to die from homicide. Validating previous studies, the highest risk for death was among people with substance abuse disorders (a nine times greater risk than among the general population). Substance use added to other psychiatric conditions was lethal. Those with personality disorders had a three times greater risk than the general population of death by homicide, followed by depression (2.6 times greater), anxiety disorders (2.2 times greater), and schizophrenia (1.8 times greater). Other risk factors for death by homicide among the mentally ill were being male, being unmarried, and having a low socioeconomic status.

The Implications for Families

In most cases, when mentally ill people are compliant with their medication and are avoiding substances, the risk for violence against their families is low. However, if the individual stops taking his psychiatric medication and starts using substances, the risk for violence escalates. This means that families should encourage medication compliance and regular visits to their psychiatrist. Substance-abusing adult children should be encouraged to attend meetings of Alcoholics Anonymous or Narcotics Anonymous and take other steps to resolve their substance issues. If the adult child refuses to comply with treatment, it may not be possible for the family to co-reside with their son or daughter anymore, because of the escalated risk of violence.

There are many reasons why people with mental illness are more likely to be victimized or even murdered. Chronic mental illness is associated with a downward social drift and the mentally ill are more likely to live in dangerous areas. Many lack the insight to accurately read their environment and stay clear of threatening situations. They are often socially ostracized and their lack of social options means they are more likely to find unstable and angry relationships. Parents of the mentally ill lie awake worrying about their child's social judgment, his friends, and the neighborhood in which he lives. They wonder, "What can I do to keep him out of harm's way?" Increasing evidence suggests that treating your child's underlying mental illness and substance abuse disorder is the best hope of keeping him safe.

Evidence That Treatment Decreases Criminal Behavior

Even though it seems intuitive, it is not easy to prove that psychiatric treatment decreases criminal behavior. Psychiatrists have long known that individuals with ADHD have an increased risk of entering a life of crime. About 30 to 40 percent of long-serving criminals have ADHD. Paul Lichtenstein and colleagues at the Karolinska Institute in Sweden studied the records of 25,000 people over a three-year period to see if treatment with standard stimulant medications affected their rate of criminal convictions. More than 8,000 people in the sample had ADHD; medication treatment decreased the rate of criminal convictions by 32 percent in men and 42 percent in women. The decline was observed in all crimes ranging from homicide and assault to less serious offenses.

Several factors might explain the lower rate of criminality among treated ADHD patients. The medications allow the patients to organize their lives more effectively and as a result, they were less likely to veer into destructive behavior. Crime often results from impulsive behavior, such as throwing a punch instead of walking away from a conflict or fleeing the

---

SOME WOMEN ARE ANTISOCIAL

When my daughter was seventeen, she had a major falling out with her boyfriend. He was a total degenerate, so we were pleased about the breakup. But then she told us that she had arranged for him to be beaten up with a baseball bat and that she was disappointed afterwards that he was still alive. She said that she was even more disappointed that he wasn't eating his dinner through a "straw in his belly," as she put it. The police were never involved and my daughter was happy with what she had done. My husband and I were appalled and we could not believe that she was capable of such terrible behavior. But she was.

---

police when pulling over to the curb would have been a better option. Stimulant medications decrease impulsive behavior more effectively than any other interventions. This study has broad public health implications and again emphasizes to parents the importance of psychiatric treatment for troubled adults.

SOME ADULTS ARE ANTISOCIAL—EVEN WHEN THEY'RE YOUR CHILDREN

The antisocial personality disorder (ASPD) is a lifelong condition dreaded in the psychiatric community and the criminal justice system. More common in men than women, ASPD individuals have an impoverished moral sense, a lack of conscience, and demonstrate a pattern of disregarding the rights of others. An adult with ASPD may be well aware of the basic constructs that govern communities but acts as if he is exempt from the rules. Only a small percentage of the general population has been diagnosed with ASPD, but they are overrepresented in the criminal justice system. Sometimes referred to as sociopaths or psychopaths, they can be superficially charming. Ask a person with ASPD who has murdered, raped, stolen, or otherwise caused bedlam what is the worst thing they have done in their life and you will hear, "I got caught."

The person with ASPD nearly always blames others for their folly rather than accepting any personal responsibility. Often they focus their problems on a previous life circumstance. They claim they found trouble because they were adopted or because they live in a crime-ridden city, or because they lack a high school diploma. People with ASPD are master manipulators and are skilled at convincing parents that they contributed to their child's misdeeds.

Parents who learn that their ASPD child has committed a crime are understandably dismayed by the news. They react by saying he was not "brought up that way," and they are often right. Some experts theorize that severe childhood abuse may lead to antisocial behavior, but most people who have been severely abused do not grow up to be sociopaths. In addition, some people who were never abused do grow up to become antisocial. ASPD individuals may emerge from stable households and may have successful parents and siblings. Neuroscientists are studying whether biological differences in the brains of those with ASPD might explain sociopathic behavior. At this point, it is not clear how to prevent ASPD from developing.

ASPD individuals push authorities to the limit and are the bane of judges and probation officers. As they have little insight into their deficiencies, they resist entering the mental health system. They are unsentimental figures with many victims in their wake and it is easy for society to cast them aside. The problem is that each person with ASPD is someone's son or daughter, and their parents struggle to respond appropriately.

Some general advice applies. Work to identify if your ASPD child has a concurrent psychiatric condition. Substance abuse and psychosis clearly magnify antisocial behavior. Antisocial personalities are more likely to have ADHD and impulsivity, a core feature of the condition that does not mix well with the absence of a social conscience. Treating the underlying psychiatric condition diminishes the risk of further bad behavior.

Often ASPD children victimize their parents, who may then decide that they have had enough heartache. In these cases detaching from your child is the only way to save yourself from the negative energy of ASPD. You might need to cut communications entirely. The painful process of estrangement with your adult child is explored in chapter 12.

HER SON IS A LYING THIEF AND IT HURTS

My son is twenty-six now and he is a thief. He has stolen thousands from us and then sold these items, threw them out, or simply gave them away. He has also allowed his friends to steal from us. Looking back, I still can't believe that I fell for all the lies. I can't believe that there is one of these awful people in my family, and he is my son. But it's true.

INVOLUNTARY PSYCHIATRIC COMMITMENT MAY BE NECESSARY

In some cases, a person may be declared mentally incompetent to stand trial. This might happen if the person was psychotic or under the influence of drugs when the crime was committed.

Every few years, the media reports a tragic story of a mother who has killed her young children. In 2001, Andrea Yates drowned her five children while experiencing postpartum psychosis, a recognized psychiatric condition characterized by the development of auditory hallucinations. The voices commanded Yates to harm her children as part of a delusion that by killing them she was in fact saving them. Yates had no history of violent behavior and the court ultimately ruled that she be committed to a hospital for treatment rather than to a prison for punishment.

During these tragedies there is a robust debate about the role of mental illness and criminal responsibility. Some contend that mental illness is a ruse and it is common to "fake" a psychotic disorder to avoid punishment. They believe that the "insanity defense" is overused. Opponents of this argument assert that mentally ill individuals often do not understand the consequences of their actions and are unjustly incarcerated. In fact, many times a court will order psychiatric treatment for an actively psychotic individual before they are tried in court. American courts believe that defendants must be well enough to help prepare their own defense. Even if they are initially deemed insane, once they are restored to sanity they face the same charges and prison sentence. Furthermore, the courts employ forensic experts who are not easily fooled by criminals pretending to be mentally ill. Finally, although it may be considerably safer than incarceration in a state prison, confinement to a state psychiatric hospital still represents a loss of freedom.

DECRIMINALIZING MENTAL ILLNESS

Most criminals with mental illness do not get adequate care in prison. An estimated 400,000 to 500,000 individuals with severe psychiatric disorders are incarcerated in jails and prisons. While they are incarcerated, these individuals may receive little treatment or no treatment. The American prison system is designed to punish criminals and to protect the rest of society from them. Most of the "correctional system" is not interested in prisoner rehabilitation.

If your adult child commits a crime and is mentally ill, be sure to tell his attorney so he can inform the court. As with mental health professionals, the attorney may be restricted from talking to you freely about your child's case, but this does not mean that *you* cannot talk to him. The judge can use this knowledge in meaningful ways. She can divert your psychiatrically ill child to the outpatient mental health system and make freedom contingent upon successfully complying with the terms of court-ordered treatment. More dramatically she can divert the criminally mentally ill to psychiatric treatment facilities instead of prison.

Mental health courts or drug courts are options that are available in some parts of the country. In these chambers the only defendants are individuals with mental illnesses. The trials are heard before jurors schooled in the relationship between mental illness and criminality. Some mental health courts may be limited to adjudicating misdemeanors, but their sensitivity to the phenomenon of mental illness usually results in a more humane outcome.

KEY POINTS IN THIS CHAPTER

- Treatment for ADHD may reduce the underlying impulsivity of those who commit crimes.

- Some adult children are antisocial and have lost their moral compass.

- Some states have mental health courts in which a serious mental illness is taken into account during sentencing.

- A mentally ill person may be guilty of a crime but be involuntarily committed to a psychiatric facility instead of prison.

The next chapter covers adults who are addicted to alcohol or drugs—or both.

CHAPTER 6

ALCOHOLISM AND DRUG ADDICTION

My daughter was married for seven years and she had already given birth to three sons when she suddenly started going out at night with friends without her husband and getting totally drunk to the point that the next day, she had no recollection whatsoever of what had happened to her. She actually did take herself to an inpatient facility at one point, but only stayed for one night and then checked out.

Alcohol use is a socially acceptable norm, and many people use alcohol and other substances responsibly. For example, narcotic prescription medications can save lives and marijuana use is increasingly mainstream. Too frequently however, the line between use and misuse is crossed. Substance use disorders are associated with tremendous behavioral difficulties and are a huge problem for families.

According to the Substance Abuse and Mental Health Services Administration (SAMHSA), about 17 million adults in the United States abuse or are dependent on alcohol. The National Institute on Drug Abuse (NIDA) has also identified the abuse of and dependence on prescription painkillers as a major problem. An estimated 4.5 million Americans abused or were dependent on marijuana in 2010. Heavy users of marijuana often abuse other substances.

Methamphetamine and cocaine are even more pernicious. In 2011, about 4 million people abused or depended on illicit drugs and about 2 million people abused narcotic pain relievers. Millions are dependent on both drugs and alcohol.

Substance abuse is a scourge that infects millions of American households, and your adult child may be a person with a substance abuse problem. She is one of many. But to you, she is very important.

This chapter provides information on why some people become addicted to alcohol and other drugs and offers information on the types of treatment that can help.

WHY DO PEOPLE USE DRUGS?

According to a 2010 report of the National Institute of Drug Abuse (NIDA), most people start abusing substances for four basic reasons:

- To feel good (and obtain feelings of euphoria, self-confidence, and increased energy)
- To feel better (to improve mood states or relieve anxiety)
- To do better (test better, suppress appetite)
- To please others (peer pressure and innate curiosity are common motives for adolescents to experiment)

People who want to "feel good" may select agents like cocaine, which offers a temporary sense of well-being and even euphoria. Pam reports that she snorted cocaine when she was younger because it allowed her to keep pace with her high-energy friends. Others abuse substances to seek a sensation of oblivion from what they perceive as their overwhelming problems. Anxious individuals may use alcohol to lessen their social awkwardness and to ease their hesitation at interacting with others. Students may seek stimulant medications to enhance their focus and concentration in a quest to improve their academic performance. Adolescents may experiment with substances to placate their friends or satiate their innate curiosity. Most people will walk away from their brief substance use without difficulty, but others will find the experience too compelling to forego it again. It is this group that is at increased risk for addiction.

Substance abuse can lead to serious problems. Marijuana can lower normal vigilance, sometimes to problematic levels. The daily marijuana smoker may be so relaxed that he inadvertently neglects his responsibilities, too stoned to notice when his toddler wanders out the front door into the street. Other substances may increase aggression. For example, as he gets high, a methamphetamine abuser may randomly assault a stranger with whom he was peacefully partying moments earlier. Some drinkers quickly transform into "angry drunks" and display their disinhibition in acts of ugly domestic violence.

Opioids are commonly prescribed narcotic painkiller drugs used to treat severe pain. Morphine, derived from the opium poppy, has been around for centuries and still has legitimate medical uses as well as being a drug of abuse. Synthetically derived drugs such as oxycodone, hydrocodone, and OxyContin are now widely available and they pose enormous addictive potential. In certain parts of the country, hospitals and prisons are overrun with young adults, often young mothers and other women, who are either being treated or punished for opiate use.

DEFINING THE PROBLEM

A few definitions will help throughout this chapter. Substance abuse refers to periodic misuse of a substance that leads to an inability to fulfill major obligations at work, school, or home. Substance abusers often are involved in dangerous activities, such as drunk driving, and may encounter legal problems. Their use of substances interferes with interpersonal relationships.

Substance abuse can devolve into dependency, a more extensive problem. While all drugs of abuse can lead to dependency (e.g., marijuana, opioids), it is the easiest to envision the plight of the alcoholic. Alcohol-dependent individuals require ever-increasing amounts of alcohol to achieve intoxication. If they are abruptly cut off from their supply, they have symptoms of withdrawal. Alcoholics who drink for years have difficulty cutting down the amount that they drink, and their usage interferes with their work and recreational activities. Alcohol-dependent individuals suffer many health problems as a result of their chronic exposure, which also makes preexisting problems like diabetes or obesity much worse.

Binge drinking is defined as consuming at least four drinks at a time for women or five drinks for men. During these times of intoxication, binge drinkers put themselves and those around them at great risk.

SIGNS AND INDICATORS OF A SUBSTANCE ABUSE PROBLEM

Experts agree that detecting substance abuse as early as possible helps to limit the subsequent devastation to individuals and families. But how do you know if your adult child may have developed a substance abuse condition? If she lives with you, it may be quite obvious that there is a problem, although you may not initially be able to identify the specific drug of abuse.

If you see your child only occasionally, it may be more difficult to identify the problem unless your child is clearly impaired during your encounters. Many times, adult children spend a lot of energy camouflaging their drug use. Parents are often the last to know that their child abuses marijuana or that she regularly drinks too much on weekends. In contrast, methamphetamine abuse is hard to hide. Abuse of this toxic drug leads to severe skin and dental problems and has a marked aging effect on most users. This section will help you identify possible general signs of a substance abuse issue.

Recommendations for Alcohol Consumption

With regard to drinking alcohol, the National Institute on Alcohol Abuse and Alcoholism (NIAAA) recommends that women should drink no more than one drink per day and men should limit their alcohol to no more than two drinks per day. A "drink" is defined as 5 ounces of wine or 12 ounces of beer or 1½ ounces of liquor.

Indicators of Alcohol Abuse and Dependence

Marci described her son Steven's struggle with alcohol. "When he was fourteen, we found empty beer cans in his bedroom. By the time he was in high school, we realized that he was stealing liquor from the cabinet and watering it down. I think we just did not take it seriously. We thought that he settled down after he left home."

By age twenty-two, Steve's alcohol problem was even more severe. By then, he had a devoted girlfriend who absorbed most of the burden. Steve could not hold down a job, and whatever money he made went to buying more alcohol. The girlfriend supported both of them. As Steve's dependency intensified, the two fought constantly. She insisted that Steve cut down on his drinking. He couldn't and, says Marci, "She left after staying with him longer than he deserved. Once she was no longer there, I tried to get Steve into treatment but his father could never admit how big the problem was until last year when we found him nearly dead."

Marci described a time when Steve could not get alcohol for several days. With the sudden cessation of drinking, he experienced physical and psychological withdrawal symptoms. The most severe of these symptoms is delirium tremens (DTs), a condition that includes auditory and visual hallucinations, seizures, confusion, and dangerous changes in blood pressure. "It wasn't until my husband saw him turn jaundiced [yellowed skin] and have a seizure that he admitted Steve's problem was very serious. For so many years we were naïve and turned our head away. I still have trouble believing how we missed the signs."

Indicators of Drug Abuse and Dependency (Addiction)

The signs of drug abuse or dependence are similar to those seen in alcoholism. A drug abuser may use occasionally, but he has not yet developed a physical tolerance to the drug. Conversely, the drug-dependent individual *does* have a physical tolerance and needs increasing quantities of drugs, even to feel "normal." He centers his psychic energy on acquiring and using drugs. An otherwise peaceful person may pursue criminal activities to fund their addiction.

The health risks for the drug abuser and drug addict vary with the type of drug that the individual relies upon. Cocaine speeds up the heart rate and can cause heart damage. Depressants have the opposite effect and the user of depressants seeks sedation. This type of self-regulated psychopharmacology can get complicated quickly. For example, a stimulant like cocaine may cause unwanted insomnia and the user sometimes incautiously pairs it with an anti-anxiety barbiturate. Another common combination is oxycodone and alcohol. Mixing drugs can have disastrous effects, including death.

DANGEROUS UNDER THE INFLUENCE

My son is thirty and he's a full-blown alcoholic. He has committed several DUIs and once he hit some people on motorcycles while drunk, after which he left the scene of the accident.

Risk Factors for Alcohol Abuse or Alcoholism

Not all individuals carry the same risk for developing substance use disorders, and well-established research shows that some groups are more vulnerable. They include:

- Individuals with ADHD, depression, anxiety disorders, bipolar disorder, or schizophrenia
- Those with ready and easy access to alcohol
- People with a low self-esteem
- Young adults who are pressured to drink
- Those who live in a culture in which alcohol use is considered normal
- People who have trouble with their relationships with others

Prescription Drug Abuse

It is not hard to convince young people that illicit drugs like cocaine or heroin are dangerous. These drugs usually originate in other countries and are completely unregulated with regard to their purity, and they may be adulterated with other unreported substances. There is no pretense that illicit drugs are manufactured with the user's safety in mind. On the other hand, prescription drugs are made in domestic high-tech plants and are under close scrutiny. They are usually prescribed by a physician for a specific medical reason. It is this false sense of security that has contributed to the dramatic rise of prescription drug abuse.

Some young people access anti-anxiety medications like Xanax to feel calm or meditative. ADHD medications like Adderall are used to enhance concentration and to improve academic performance even in individuals who do not have ADHD. In general, neither of these common occurrences is associated with negative or violent behavior. However, the same cannot be said of misused opioid medications. These painkillers offer to some a dreamy euphoria that is highly addictive. Ironically, this pursuit of tranquility is associated with scheming behavior.

The Cycle of Narcotic Abuse Begins

Two major routes lead to opiate abuse. Young people can be exposed to narcotics after a legitimate injury. A small percentage of them will find the unique properties of opioids to be tremendously appealing and will crave the sensation even after the pain episode has resolved.

More commonly, however, young people will plot to obtain opioids. Sometimes it starts by stealing grandpa's oxycodone. Often the first exposure comes via a friend. The addiction can develop quickly and become all-consuming.

Drug-Seeking Activities

Life for an individual who is dependent on prescription medications is treacherous. Many addicts will seek a doctor for a prescription. They quickly learn that it is not hard to obtain the first painkiller, but most doctors are reluctant to offer easy refills. Unfortunately, every city has a few uninformed or unscrupulous physicians who accede to these requests and their names circulate among addicts.

Some adults go from one emergency room to another with fictitious physical complaints to score a prescription. Most ER doctors are suspicious of nebulous complaints like recurrent headaches. Also, the use of electronic medical records has made this practice less popular. In addition, most states now have prescription monitoring laws that require pharmacists to report prescribed narcotics to a central authority. Thus, if one person convinces multiple doctors to write prescriptions for narcotics, the surveillance system will flag this pattern.

Once exposed to opioids, some patients experience considerable difficulty giving up the perceived benefits of these drugs. Desperate antisocial behaviors emerge. It is not uncommon for the addict to injure himself purposefully to create a pain condition that requires treatment. He may forge prescriptions or resort to stealing from pharmacies. Pain medications are available on the street but they are expensive, the supply is inconsistent, and the criminal penalties are harsh.

WHY SOME INDIVIDUALS ARE PRONE TO ADDICTION AND OTHERS ARE NOT: A COMPLEX QUESTION

It's often hard to know why some patients can take narcotics after an injury and then never take them again once they recover. In a similar way, some people can take one alcoholic drink and stop, while for others, that first drink is a gateway to alcohol abuse and alcoholism. Some experts believe that the problem is largely driven by a genetic predisposition to addictive behavior, and they cite the fact that addictions tend to run in families. Others see the problem as largely environmental. For example, you can be pressured to use by friends or you can choose friends who use.

If Psychiatric Problems Are Also Present

In many cases of substance abuse and dependence, the individual has an underlying psychiatric disorder. Common conditions include attention-deficit hyperactivity disorder (ADHD), depression, and generalized anxiety disorder. The adult child may also develop a personality disorder, such as borderline personality disorder or antisocial personality disorder. Many times these conditions occur concurrently.

While each psychiatric disorder is unique, with different brain chemical abnormalities that are responsive to different medications, anxiety and depression are common among a wide range of disorders. Those who suffer often find that alcohol and other drugs temporarily neutralize their intense psychological discomfort. Almost always, this method of self-treatment complicates the underlying illness. Understanding substance abuse as a means to self-medicate psychological pain is a medically valid and humane way of viewing addiction.

"My mind raced all the time," Cheryl recalls. "I could not shut it off. I worried about everything. If there were good things in my life, I could not stop thinking how to keep them good. When bad things happened, I focused everything on how to make things different. I was miserable when I finished top in my law school, I was miserable when my family was young and innocent. I was miserable when my marriage fell apart. The only respite I got was from marijuana. At least with marijuana, I could sleep a few hours."

Cheryl continues, "As my kids got older, I did not want to smoke in front of them and when my own son got a DUI, I found it harder to continue smoking. As I was trying to get him help, he was diagnosed with panic disorder and obsessive-compulsive disorder. I realized immediately that I had the same conditions. After a few months of treatment, I felt better. My sleep improved on these medications and I no longer felt preoccupied with smoking grass. I hope my son will agree to treatment so that he gets the same benefit."

TIPS FOR PARENTS

- Don't openly store your drugs or alcohol.
- Don't serve alcohol at family functions. It's too tempting.
- Don't give up on treatment. It may take several attempts.

Don't Openly Store Your Drugs or Alcohol

It's far too much temptation for the substance abuser if you leave your own alcohol or drugs openly displayed. Lock up both drugs and alcohol. You should also get rid of all old narcotics. The FDA recommends that you get rid of unused narcotics by participating in programs in which the city or county offers take-back drug days for such drugs to be disposed of by local law enforcement agencies. If this option is not available and there are no disposal directions on the drug packaging, then the drug should be taken from the prescription bottle and put in a container of used kitty litter or coffee grounds, to disguise and also discourage any reuse.

Remove the labels with your name and other information on it from the now-empty drug containers and tear them up so that no one can gain information about your pharmacy account or can gain access to your prescription information.

Don't Serve Alcohol at Family Functions

Hold off the alcohol at family events when your adult child who is an alcoholic is present. Instead, serve nonalcoholic drinks, juice, water, or soda. Some relatives may object, but they'll get by.

Don't Give Up on Treatment

Hopefully the first time your adult child receives treatment will be the last time she needs it. But people with substance abuse often relapse, and this may also happen with your child. It's disappointing but do not give up.

TREATMENT OF SUBSTANCE DEPENDENCE

Like a noxious vapor in a closed room, alcoholism and substance use permeate every aspect of life. The health risks include damage to the liver and the pancreas and gastrointestinal cancers. The behaviors associated with substance use, depression, and suicide can tear a family apart. Unfortunately, many substance abusers do not acknowledge that they have a problem, let alone that they need to be part of the solution. As a result, trying to convince your adult child to get treatment can be an uphill battle. Sustaining that recovery can be remarkably frustrating for families. Keep in mind that the mere act of agreeing to treatment is a major milestone for a person who is addicted to a substance.

Self-Help Groups for People with Alcoholism and Substance Use Disorders

The good news is that a number of different treatments can work. Self-help groups play a paramount role for all types of substance abuse. In some cases individual psychotherapy is needed. If these efforts fail, residential treatment is required. Medications can also play a supportive role in therapy. Some medications decrease alcohol and opioid cravings, while others are designed to make the person physically ill if they drink alcohol within days of taking the pill. Medications can indirectly combat substance abuse (as seen in Cheryl's story) by addressing the underlying psychiatric conditions that propel the abuse.

The first lines of treatment are self-help groups, and the best known is Alcoholics Anonymous. Alcoholics Anonymous (AA) stresses a complete avoidance of all alcohol. The abstinence message is reinforced by peer support and with regular attendance at daily meetings. Addicts who are newly in recovery are paired with sober sponsors. AA meetings are free to attend and take place daily in every major city throughout the world. AA subscribes to a twelve-step process of abstinence. The first step is the acknowledgment that the individual has lost control over his use of alcohol. Narcotics Anonymous (NA) and related self-help programs incorporate similar twelve-step principles to aid people who are drug addicted. NA-centered programs are useful for marijuana and stimulant abuse disorders.

Not all adults accept self-help programs. Some object to the apparent spiritual nature of twelve-step programs, although the "higher power" to which the individual surrenders can signify whatever the individual wishes and does not need to be a religious icon. In large cities, twelve-step programs that make no reference to God thrive. Other less well-known self-help groups include Women for Sobriety, an organization for women with alcohol dependency and other forms of addiction (women forsobriety.org); Secular Organizations for Sobriety (cfiwest.org/sos/index.htm), run by founder Jim Christopher; and Smart Recovery (smartrecovery.org).

Outpatient Therapy Treatment

For others, self-help groups or group therapy can feel like an invasion of privacy. In these situations individual psychotherapy may be a helpful alternative. For example, cognitive-behavioral therapy (CBT) is a well-regarded form of individual therapy used with this population. With CBT, the individual is trained to identify and then challenge their irrational and self-defeating thoughts, replacing them with more rational and positive thoughts. Read more about CBT in chapter 9.

Some therapists use *motivational interviewing*, in which the therapist helps the client find her own personal reasons for staying off alcohol and/or drugs. The theory is that the motivation for change must come from within. If a therapist lectures his young patient on the evils of substances, it is tempting for the patient to refuse or resist these conclusions because he does not own them. The theory behind motivational interviewing is that if the patient generates the reasons for avoiding drugs and alcohol himself, then he is less likely to waste time and energy trying to prove the therapist wrong.

QUESTIONS TO ASK TREATMENT FACILITIES

Before your child is admitted to a local treatment facility, it is ideal to visit, observe, and inquire about specific issues.

1. Does the program accept the individual's insurance? If not, will they work with the individual or the family on creating a payment plan or identifying another means of payment?
2. Is the program operated by state-accredited and licensed professionals?
3. Is the facility well organized and clean?
4. Does the program offer the full range of services needed by an individual, such as medical care and vocational services?
5. Does the program offer age-, gender-, and culturally appropriate activities for residents?
6. Are aftercare services provided and encouraged?
7. Is the treatment plan assessed on an ongoing basis to ensure it meets the changing needs of the individual?
8. Does the program use strategies to keep individuals in longer-term treatment, thus increasing the likelihood of success?
9. Does the program offer individual and group counseling?
10. Does the program offer medication as part of the regimen, if appropriate?
11. Is there an ongoing monitoring of potential relapse, to aid in guiding patients back to abstinence for the substance to which they are addicted?
12. Does the program offer services to family members to ensure they understand both addiction and the recovery process, so that they are better able to help the recovering person?

Inpatient Facilities for Treatment

Unfortunately, outpatient treatment does not always yield the desired result of sobriety, and more intensive treatment settings are often needed to treat addiction. Inpatient substance abuse facilities may provide services for weeks and residential units for months or longer. Inpatient substance abuse treatment is costly, and in recent years insurance companies have made it increasingly difficult to secure this form of treatment. But in certain cases nothing else works. Inpatient treatment offers obvious advantages. First, having a physical barrier between the patient and any available substances of abuse serves to decrease the likelihood of a relapse. Secondly, inpatient units allow for regular family meetings and treating staff can arrange an efficient transition to an outpatient treatment plan.

Most importantly, the inpatient treatment team can observe the patient when she is substance-free and this can clarify whether an underly-

---

ENTERING RESIDENTIAL TREATMENT FOR ALCOHOL OR DRUG ADDICTION

Kai credits his wife's diligence in finding an appropriate treatment center for their son's recovery. David, now twenty-three, developed an addiction to methamphetamine when he returned from service in Afghanistan. At first, he refused to go to the local VA treatment clinic because he feared that treatment within the system would interfere with his plan to re-enlist. He was also distrustful of local civilian clinics. A year and a half of family misery followed.

Kai reported, "My wife found a treatment center in Florida that had a specialized program for methamphetamine treatment." He says that David went to this center and the treatment clicked for him. David started as an inpatient and found camaraderie in group therapy. He was started on antidepressant medications. As David made progress, he was able to transition to an apartment nearby with other young men also in recovery. Kai said, "I think the warm weather and the community living helped him enormously. The facility arranged for family therapy. Fortunately, our insurance paid for the majority of his care. After three months, David was able to stabilize and regain his trust. When he returned home, David felt more comfortable at the VA clinic. He is doing very well."

ing psychiatric diagnosis exists. For instance, if a patient is suffering from both depression and alcohol dependency, the depression may be overlooked and remain untreated until the substance abuse layer is peeled away. Once identified, the depression can be treated.

Many larger cities have several sophisticated inpatient facilities. It is best to enter a program led by a psychiatrist so that the substance abuse and other underlying psychiatric issues can be identified and treated. Programs that simply focus on abstinence and sobriety are inadequate. If your child does not find success at local treatment facilities, families may consider national centers like the Brighton Hospital in Brighton, Michigan, or Hazelden in ten cities nationwide in Florida, Illinois, Minnesota, New York, and Oregon (hazelden.org). If your child does not find success at local treatment facilities, families may consider national centers like the Brighton, Michigan, or Hazelden in ten cities nationwide in Florida, Illinois, Minnesota, New York, and Oregon (hazelden.org). The cost and getting to these excellent facilities can be obstacles, but they are often worth the investment.

Follow-Up after Discharge Is Important

Once your child has been discharged from an inpatient treatment facility, then outpatient follow-up with a treatment team is necessary to minimize the risk of a relapse. The best program will have an affiliated outpatient unit; in this circumstance the philosophy of the inpatient unit carries over. Unfortunately, relapses are common, even for the most dedicated patients treated in the most advanced programs. As mentioned earlier, twelve-step programs such as Alcoholics Anonymous or Narcotics Anonymous should be a part of the outpatient treatment plan.

Treatment for the Family

Living with active substance abusers can be anxiety provoking, heart wrenching, and infuriating—all at the same time. Parents witness their children making terrible choices and then paying the consequences for these decisions. Many families turn to Al-Anon, a support group for the families of alcoholics. Here families meet regularly and support one another, and it has become a community that lessens the sense of loneliness that each family inevitably has. What has worked for one family may also help another family. Families that are new to the problems are comforted by families that have struggled longer, and both groups find the support process to be therapeutic.

Community resources can be shared during these meetings, including which mental health professionals and facilities in the area may specialize in substance abuse treatment.

MEDICATIONS FOR SUBSTANCE ABUSE/DEPENDENCY

The best way of becoming clean and sober is to stop drinking (or using drugs). Alas, this is easy to say and very difficult to accomplish for most people who are substance-dependent.

Some medications are designed to minimize the withdrawal symptoms that occur immediately after stopping the offending substance. Others directly curb cravings for drugs or make alcohol use highly unappealing.

Medications Used in Detoxifications

Individuals may abuse drugs ranging from alcohol to cocaine and prescription narcotics. The specific method of treatment for each of these addictions differs but a major obstacle for all substance abusers is the profound discomfort associated with the first few days of abstinence. Detoxification refers to the withdrawal from the addicting drug. Inpatient and outpatient facilities monitor the patient's health as she detoxifies from drugs and alcohol. Ideally, detoxification is performed under a physician's care because complications often arise. Benzodiazepines (lorazepam, clonazepam) are commonly used for alcohol withdrawal to reduce the likelihood of seizures and ease the symptoms of agitation, changes in pulse and blood pressure, and altered thought processes. Particular care must accompany the timing of the detoxification medications because the simultaneous use of benzodiazepine medications and alcohol can be dangerous. Some physicians believe that anticonvulsant medications (topiramate, carbamazepine) are superior to benzodiazepines for alcohol detoxification. Clonidine, a medication also used to treat high blood pressure, is commonly used for opioid withdrawal.

An alternative school of thought is that withdrawal should be fully experienced by addicts. Physicians with this viewpoint believe that the promise of a medication-cushioned withdrawal makes the psychological and physical cost of relapse too low and serves to reinforce the underlying drug-abusing behavior. Your adult child has about an even chance of encountering a doctor who subscribes to the philosophy of using medications to ease withdrawal or one who is opposed to such use.

Once detoxification is complete, a number of medications are available to decrease relapses. The medications can be taken over months and years and are most helpful when used with psychosocial therapies. See the chart on page 101 for a summary of medications used to treat alcoholism and opioid dependence.

Medications Used in Treatment

After detoxification occurs (with or without the help of medications), medications such as disulfiram, naltrexone, methadone, and other medications help people to get off and stay off alcohol and the drugs to which they were addicted.

Disulfiram

Disulfiram, which is usually known by the trade name Antabuse, inactivates an enzyme needed to break down alcohol and it is used to treat alcoholics. As a result, even small quantities of ingested alcohol are transformed into a chemical that causes severe nausea and vomiting. If your child drinks within forty-eight hours of taking Antabuse, he will pay an uncomfortable toll.

This aversive method is most helpful for impulsive drinking. Disulfiram needs to be taken daily and under most circumstances has no effect. But if alcohol is consumed, the effects are profoundly unpleasant, so many people are fearful of taking the medication or do not stick with it for long periods.

Disulfiram treatment may be ordered by a court as a part of a comprehensive compulsory treatment plan that includes individual and group therapy. The medication can be taken at AA meetings and compliance can be recorded for the court. It also allows parents to watch their child take the medication in the morning to ensure that they will not drink at night.

Medications Used to Treat Substance Dependency

Generic Name of Drug (Brand Name)	For Alcohol Treatment?	For Treatment of Opioid Dependency?	Side Effects of Drug	Key Benefits	Key Problems
Disulfiram (Antabuse)	Yes	No	Stops the body's ability to break down alcohol. Causes severe nausea and vomiting even with small amounts of alcohol. May also cause anxiety and fatigue. Patients may experience a metallic taste in the mouth.	Very effective when taken.	Can cause rapid heartbeat and sweating if patient drinks alcohol. May also lead to coronary artery disease. Many patients refuse to take the drug unless it is court-ordered.
Methadone	No	Yes	Also used by some doctors for pain management, although some physicians are not aware of potential risks and possible drug interactions. The FDA says that methadone should *not* be the first drug of choice for those with severe pain. Is potentially an addictive drug.	Effective and helps to prevent opioid addicts from seeking injected drugs on the street.	Can be addicting if patient takes more than the prescribed dosage. It is also an opioid and should not be combined with other opioids.
Acamprosate (Campral)	Yes	No	May cause sleepiness and diarrhea.	Increases number of alcohol-free days.	Rarely, may lead to thoughts of suicide and should be avoided in those with past suicidal attempts or with depression.
Naltrexone (Depade, ReVia); injectable naltrexone (Vivitrol)	Yes	Yes	Reduces craving for alcohol or opioids.	May help with alcoholism or opioid addiction.	Should not be used if person has liver or kidney disease or needs to take other opioids.
Buprenorphine (Subutex) and buprenorphine/naloxone (Suboxone)	No	Yes	Headaches, nausea, mood swings, difficulty sleeping and sweating. Can be addictive if misused.	May decrease the craving for opioids.	May cause insomnia, headache, sweating, and nausea. These drugs are sometimes abused.

Disulfiram is not indicated in individuals with heart disease and should be used only with caution in people with a history of diabetes or kidney disease. Disulfiram reacts with some drugs, particularly warfarin (Coumadin), phenytoin (Dilantin), and over-the-counter drugs that contain alcohol. If disulfiram is being considered for treatment, the person should have a blood test of their liver function beforehand to ensure that no liver disease is currently present.

Naltrexone and Vivitrol

For many years, doctors have used naltrexone and naloxone. Both are opiate blockers that decrease the action of the pleasure centers of the brain. As a result, the physiological "high" associated with substances of abuse is less intensely registered. The National Institute of Alcohol Abuse and Alcoholism (NIAAA) reports that oral naltrexone (Depade, ReVia) decreases the risk for relapse by about a third when a patient is in the first three months of treatment. An injectable extended-release form of naltrexone can be administered monthly. Vivitrol has been shown specifically to decrease the number of serious drinking days. Insurance companies are increasingly offering coverage for this monthly injectable medication.

Campral

Acamprosate (Campral) is another medication shown in clinical trials to promote sobriety. The medication decreases craving for alcohol and thus helps to end drinking, but it needs to be taken three times daily. Even when patients are regularly reminded that sobriety is an hour-to-hour proposition, the demands of this schedule are hard to maintain, and the early promise of this drug has not been realized. Campral comes in an oral tablet form. Kidney function should be assessed before starting the medication and throughout treatment.

Methadone

Methadone maintenance therapy has been used since the 1960s to treat heroin and prescription opioid addiction. Methadone, like heroin, is an opioid, but it is long-acting and it is administered by mouth rather than by needle. A primary advantage of methadone maintenance is that heroin addicts are able to avoid sharing contaminated needles. As a result they are much less likely to transmit bloodborne diseases such as the human immunodeficiency virus (HIV) or hepatitis.

In recent years, methadone clinics have become less popular. Voices in the substance abuse treatment community argue that although methadone is safer than heroin, it remains an addictive drug. Some politicians and the Food and Drug Administration (FDA) have become disenchanted with methadone, because methadone clinics are expensive to operate, tend to maintain rather than halt opioid use, and methadone clinics may also have an interest in extending the length of treatment. Another problem is that for some drug-dependent patients, the long-acting effects of methadone are preferred over the use of heroin and the easy access via a maintenance clinic gives them little incentive to quit opioids altogether. Furthermore, methadone patients may continue to use alcohol, and the combination of both substances can be fatal.

Methadone is still used by pain management doctors for chronic non-cancerous pain, such as severe back pain or frequent headaches. The Centers for Disease Control and Prevention (CDC) reports that more than 4 million prescriptions of methadone for pain management were written in 2009. Recent CDC reports suggest that methadone may not be very helpful for these health problems and that long-term use may be dangerous. Although methadone represented only about 5 percent of all prescribed opioids in 2009, about 30 percent of opioid-related deaths that year were associated with methadone. The fact that methadone is frequently diverted to other addicts may contribute to this alarming number of deaths.

Bupenorphine

The current standard medication therapy for treating opioid dependency is buprenorphine (Subutex) or buprenorphine combined with naloxone (Suboxone). Buprenorphine carries a lower risk for addiction than other opioids such as oxycodone. When combined with an opiate receptor blocker, the patient receives a muted high. When this dosage is slowly reduced, the transition to becoming free of opioids is much easier to tolerate.

Suboxone has been approved by the FDA for office-based treatment of opioid addiction by physicians with specialized training. Subutex may be given in the early stages of detoxification while Suboxone is used during the maintenance phase of the treatment.

The successful plan demands that the physician and patient determine a titration schedule (tapering down the medication) and stick to it, acknowledging in advance that each dose reduction will be temporarily distressing to the patient. Making the transition from pure opioid to Suboxone represents progress, but complete cessation of opiates and opiate treatment agents is the intended goal.

These drugs can be given by prescription and they are less tightly controlled than with other opiate dependency treatments. Suboxone comes in the form of a thin film that dissolves rapidly in the mouth. Side effects may include headaches, sweating, nausea, mood swings, and insomnia. Like other opiates, Suboxone may cause a person to have trouble breathing if the medication is taken with alcohol or other depressant medications.

WHAT YOU CAN AND CANNOT DO ABOUT YOUR CHILD'S SUBSTANCE ABUSE PROBLEM

As a parent of an adult child with a substance abuse or dependence issue, of course you want to help your child if you can. It's important to know that there are some things you can do to help and others that are not so helpful. The chart on page 105 offers you some suggestions.

Convincing Your Adult Child to Get Help

You want to help your adult child become clean and sober. Sometimes this goal is achieved quickly, but more often, several attempts are needed to get it right. Frequently your child is an unwilling participant or is reluctant because of her past treatment failures. A solid strategy is to schedule a family meeting with your child's permission. Ideally this occurs at a counselor's office, although the family may need to stage the discussion alone if a counselor is not in the picture. At such a meeting, family members express their concern at the ongoing substance use and encourage their

What You Can and Cannot Do to Help Your Child
with Substance Abuse Issues

What You Can Do	What You Cannot Do
Recommend your adult child go to meetings of Alcoholics Anonymous, Narcotics Anonymous, or other self-help groups.	Force your child to attend a self-help group. (You can, however, make it a condition of living in your home.)
Recommend your child seek medical treatment for substance issues.	Compel your child to seek treatment. (Unless it is a condition of living at your home.)
Learn about your child's problem.	Cure your child.
Stage an intervention to encourage inpatient treatment.	Compel your child to go to treatment after an intervention

loved one to pursue the next level of treatment. "This is the time to consider a medication, or you need to sign yourself into a treatment center," are common refrains heard at these meetings.

Sometimes a more dramatic effort is required. "Interventions" have become grist for the reality show mill, and many television viewers have seen several memorable examples. Effective interventions are highly orchestrated meetings where family and friends confront the adult child (or other person) about the negative impact of their substance abuse. The goal is for the ill person to agree to enter treatment directly after the intervention. A mental health professional trusted by your child should lead the intervention. It's important to remember that interventions are a high-stakes tactic that can backfire.

Steps in an Intervention

The Mayo Clinic outlines key steps for an intervention. First, the intervention should be planned with a mental health professional who is both trained and experienced in interventions. An appropriate inpatient treatment facility with specific expertise with your child's type of addiction (i.e., prescription drugs, alcohol, cross-addiction) should be chosen with input from the therapist.

Next, the team members must be identified and recruited. Team members generally include family members and friends, hopefully all united in their commitment to treatment. They must be willing to speak candidly to your child about the emotional pain that the addict has caused them. For example, Linda recalls that in a meeting prior to an intervention for her older brother Robert, she decided to tell him how much she resented that he was intoxicated at her wedding ceremony. Robert's mother seethed that he did not show up for his grandfather's funeral because he was drunk, and she realized that she needed to let him know of her resentment. Interventions become the forum to convey these feelings.

At these pre-intervention meetings, team members need to identify what consequences they are willing to enforce should your child refuse the overture for treatment. For leverage, families can plan to withhold money or lodging or refuse to allow their adult child to see certain family members. Linda recalls making the decision that Robert could not see her year-old daughter until he got clean. "I am not used to making threats, but I had to protect him and protect my family," said Linda.

Individual members should write down ahead of time what they plan to say when the intervention occurs, so they don't forget in the heat of the moment.

Intervention Day

On the day of the intervention, your child is asked by a member to go to the site. She often will guess the agenda when she sees key people in her life glumly sitting together. Don't be surprised if she asks to leave before the meeting starts, but usually the force of so many familiar faces keeps her there.

The intervention starts with the leader expressing their love and the group's desire that more extensive treatment take place. Each member will then get a chance to speak. The consequences of not acting will be clearly outlined.

Does Intervention Work?

According to Copello and colleagues there is "robust evidence" that family interventions work for alcohol or drug dependence. However, it is important to understand that interventions can go either way. In the best case, the person will agree to seek treatment immediately.

Another possible outcome is that the person will become angry, continue to deny her addiction, and walk out. Even if this occurs, the seed has been planted and your child may become more amenable to treatment down the line. In the worst case, the adult child refuses help, the family's actions are enacted without impact, and a permanent break occurs in the family. Your child continues to abuse substances, but now without family contact.

KEY POINTS IN THIS CHAPTER

- Alcoholics and other addicts exhibit similar symptoms, such as the centering of their lives on using the substance and finding more.

- Some medications can ease the detoxification from alcohol or drugs and help people stay off these substances. But some doctors prefer to withhold these medications.

- People with substance abuse issues often have psychiatric conditions that need to be treated as well.

- An intervention may encourage your child to receive inpatient treatment, but it requires careful planning and does not always work.

The next chapter describes psychiatric problems that often contribute to serious behavioral issues.

CHAPTER 7
OTHER PSYCHIATRIC PROBLEMS

My daughter is thirty and she lives with me. She has both bipolar disorder and anxiety and she's also an addict who won't get treatment. She hates her life, and so often wishes that she would die. She has tried to commit suicide numerous times, and she also constantly uses marijuana and opiates to numb her severe emotional pain. It's very hard to witness my daughter suffering so much.

Earlier chapters have emphasized that psychiatric illnesses are at the core of much problem behavior, and also that parenting a troubled adult child tests families on a daily basis. Families are often extremely frustrated by their child's behavior and confused about how best to respond.

Parents of troubled adult children seek to understand the limitations imposed by their child's illness and balance that knowledge with realistic expectations. Parents tell me frequently that "I want to help my child, but I do not want to enable him." They are fearful that their well-meaning actions are counterproductive and might make a bad situation even worse and say, "If I help my twenty-six-year-old son with rent this month, then he will expect the same next month." On the other hand, they are equally concerned that if they withhold too much, their child will flounder. These families remark, "If I don't make sure she gets her morning medications, she spends a wasted day in bed."

Of course, each case is unique and every family responds as best they can. Your troubled adult child did not come with an instruction manual and no website offers an easy recipe for parenting. As such, the premise of this chapter is that it is important to define and understand the common psychiatric conditions that might befall your child so your family can strike the delicate balance between helping and hindering.

Certainly not all problematic behavior results from mental illness, and folklore teaches that it is not easy, even for a forensic psychiatrist, to tell whether a patient is "plain bad" or is mentally ill. Certain psychiatric conditions occur frequently in the young adult population. Chapter 6 focuses on substance use disorders. This chapter covers the full array of anxiety disorders and mood disorders (including depression and bipolar disorder), as well as other disorders that may have a devastating impact.

Schizophrenia is a devastating psychotic disease affecting both thought and behavior that causes physical alterations in the brain. A growing body of evidence suggests that the brains of patients with obsessive-compulsive disorder and major depressive disorder function in characteristic patterns. There is less evidence that personality disorders are brain-based, which neither buoys nor consoles the parents of children with borderline or antisocial personality disorder.

We extend the discussion of psychiatric disorders to attention-deficit hyperactivity disorder (ADHD). ADHD is not limited to children: It is one of the most treatable conditions afflicting young adults and it is commonly misidentified and undertreated.

In addition, this chapter provides information on intermittent explosive disorder (IED), a condition of unpredictable outbursts that wreaks havoc with families, and mild autism spectrum disorder (formerly known as Asperger's syndrome). Like all psychiatric conditions, mild autism spectrum disorder has been a part of the human condition since day one, but only recently have experts wrestled with the science behind it and the impact that this condition has on families.

Key elements of these disorders and their treatments are summarized in the chart on page 124.

ANXIETY DISORDERS

The waiting rooms of many therapists are filled with patients who are diagnosed with one or more anxiety disorders. Generalized anxiety disorder (GAD), panic disorder, obsessive-compulsive disorder (OCD), and specific phobias (such as fears of contamination or the fear of having blood drawn) might sound trite to the casual observer, but these disorders can be disabling. Post-traumatic stress disorder (PTSD) is an anxiety disorder that receives considerable attention because of its high prevalence in military veterans.

These anxiety disorders are all very real, and they cause the individual great suffering. Anxiety disorders severely interfere with daily functioning, rendering the patient unable to live a normal life. Most suffer quietly unless they receive treatment. Parents are called upon, sometimes by default, because their adult child has nowhere else to turn.

Generalized Anxiety Disorder

The Diagnostic and Statistical Manual (DSM-5), the major publication of the American Psychiatric Association, published in 2013, describes the key features of all psychiatric diagnoses. Anxiety disorders can stand alone, but frequently a patient will have more than one condition.

Generalized anxiety disorder is a condition of severe and persistent worry. People with GAD worry incessantly about their health, their work, their family, and sometimes about the banal aspects of their daily lives. Most realize that their worrying is excessive, but recognition alone does not make the anxiety any easier to control. About 3 percent of the adult population in the United States has GAD, and at least a third have severe symptoms. About twice as many women as men suffer from GAD. The highest risk of onset is between childhood and middle age, although the symptoms can surface at any age.

Panic Disorder

Individuals with panic disorder endure repeated anxiety attacks that are manifested by a feeling of imminent disaster. Intense fear and anxiety are the overwhelming psychological sensations of panic attacks, but the accompanying physical symptoms are particularly troublesome. During a panic attack, people develop a racing pulse, difficulty breathing, profuse perspiration, chest and stomach pain, and numbness and tingling throughout the body, making them feel doomed. In the United States, about 2.7 percent of adults have panic disorder and about half of them

(1.2 percent of adults) have severe symptoms. The average age of the onset of panic disorder is twenty-four, according to the NIMH.

Every human has the ability to panic, and sometimes it is an appropriate physiological response. If you had a gun jammed in your back by an attacker demanding your wallet, it would make sense for your heart to pound and your breathing to speed up. Your body is preparing to flee to safety. The problem is that with a panic attack, this response can occur out of the blue, even when no discernible threat is present. These attacks can occur during stressful life circumstances as well as during periods of calm. When individuals experience panic attacks, they fear that they are in mortal danger. They frequently end up in hospital emergency rooms, convinced that they are having a heart attack or a stroke.

It is the task of the physician to make sure that her panic disorder patient is not having a life-threatening event (most young people do not have heart attacks and certainly not several times a month), but once this is established, it is important to offer reassurance. "You are healthy, but your body is tricking you into a reaction to a threat that does not exist." This simple explanation can be highly therapeutic to the panic sufferer. Patients who do not receive this reassurance may live for years in fear that death is imminent.

Obsessive-Compulsive Disorder (OCD)

Obsessive-compulsive disorder is an anxiety disorder in which the individual has constant intrusive thoughts (obsessions), as well as frequent repetitive behaviors (compulsions). There are many variations of this condition, and sometimes obsessions are more troubling than compulsions or vice versa.

In one recent case, a young mother could not shake the obsessive thought that she was going to smother her young children. Nothing could be further from the truth, but reassurance from her family and her doctor that this would never happen did not suppress her worry. She found that washing her hands and counting by twelves gave her temporary relief from the inescapable images. But soon the compulsive cleaning rituals extended on for hours and the endless counting rendered her incapable of doing much else. According to the National Institute of Mental Health, about 1 percent of the population suffers from OCD, half of whom suffer severely. The average age of the onset of OCD is nineteen.

It is unknown what causes OCD. Brain imaging reveals an endless loop of nonproductive activity. OCD is treated with antidepressant medications and cognitive-behavioral therapy (CBT), as well as exposure and response prevention therapy. For example, the young mother was instructed *not* to count or wash her hands. She was then to observe that absent her rituals, no disaster occurred (her children were unharmed). The repetitive but pragmatic therapy eventually alleviated her debilitating worry.

Post-Traumatic Stress Disorder (PTSD)

Post-traumatic stress disorder stems from exposure to severe trauma such as a combat experience, rape, or a catastrophic event (e.g., being stranded underground without hope of being found). According to the NIMH, about 3.5 percent of the adult population suffers from PTSD, with an average age of the onset of the disorder occurring in the early twenties.

Individuals with PTSD experience flashbacks as if they were reliving the trauma but in real time. In other words, these flashbacks are not static memories, but instead are experienced as if the person is reliving the initial trauma. For example, soldiers may have flashbacks of a bloody firefight while flood victims may flashback to their desperate experience with rising waters and nowhere to flee. Victims of childhood sexual abuse flashback to memories when they were shamed or humiliated sexually by another person. Flashbacks are accompanied by a powerful surge of anxiety and a sense of shame or grief.

Individuals with PTSD also often suffer from recurrent negative thoughts, insomnia, and nightmares. The individual may be very tense, and may avoid places and objects that remind him of the initial trauma. They may also experience hyperarousal, or becoming very easily startled. For example, the veteran with PTSD may dive for cover if he hears a car backfire, even if the original firefight happened to him years earlier. PTSD is a chronic anxiety disorder, although the person may not exhibit any symptoms for weeks or months after the initial traumatizing event. Among

PTSD victims, outbursts of anger are common; these are intensified if alcohol is used.

Treatment of Anxiety Disorders

Generalized anxiety disorder is treated with therapy and with medications. The first-line treatments for GAD are antidepressant medications. Anti-anxiety medications are also commonly used, particularly those in the benzodiazepine class, such as clonazepam (Klonopin) and alprazolam (Xanax). These medications are drugs controlled by the Drug Enforcement Administration (DEA), because they have the potential to be misused. Drugs known as atypical antipsychotics in low doses can also be helpful in severe cases of GAD.

Panic disorder is treated with psychotherapy and antidepressant medications. Anti-anxiety drugs, particularly lorazepam (Ativan) and alprazolam (Xanax), help in the early stages of recovery, and also may be useful over long periods of time. Beta blocker medications such as propranolol (Inderal) help control the pounding heart, dizziness, and severe perspiring that accompany panic attacks, although they are not effective at reducing core anxiety.

OCD is treated with antidepressants such as sertraline (Zoloft) and paroxetine (Paxil), medications that are also used in PTSD treatment. Both conditions respond to psychotherapy as well. For OCD, cognitive behavioral therapy is recommended. More examples of this technique are included in chapter 9.

Exposure therapy also works well in PTSD. With this approach, patients are gradually exposed to an anxiety-provoking situation. For example, a rape victim suffering from PTSD initially may not leave her home or socialize with non–family members. She instinctively will avoid returning to the place where she was raped. A seasoned therapist will design a plan of gradual exposure. At first, she is encouraged to venture out of her home to test the waters. The patient soon discovers that the fear is worse than the actual threat and then becomes ready for the next step. She may be instructed to go to a restaurant, first with her family and then alone. A graduation exercise will be to return to the crime scene so as to demystify the trauma. With consistent and expanding exposure work, her freedom to move about can be fully restored.

LIVING WITH AN ADULT CHILD
WITH AN ANXIETY DISORDER

Jenny was twenty-four years old when she came to my office. Back in middle school, Jenny was diagnosed with OCD. Her anxiety revolved around an intense fear of becoming contaminated by germs. This unrealistic fear prevented her from leaving her house, and she retreated from her friends and other social interactions. Jenny's reserve was in sharp contrast to the outgoing nature of her older brother, who was president of the student council and was comfortable with all types of people.

By her late teens, Jenny had partially recovered, and she decided to enter the local university. Her adjustment to dormitory life went well at first, until she attended a fraternity party with several friends. At the party, Jenny became intoxicated and disinhibited. A young man whom she knew casually brought her back to her dorm. The next week, pictures of Jenny appearing drunk and barely clothed were posted by others on Facebook. She barely remembered the episode and was too afraid to tell anyone.

But the episode proved devastating to Jenny, who was very embarrassed by the online photos and stunned by the reaction of the people in her dormitory. The jokes about her "slutty" behavior were not intended to humiliate Jenny, but they did.

The following week, Jenny's roommate discovered that Jenny had stopped going to class or doing her work. She also developed panic attacks. The panic attacks would hit several times a week and they disabled her. Jenny also developed insomnia and she suffered from flashbacks of the fraternity party and the aftermath.

Jenny told her parents what happened and how bad she felt. Finding little help on campus, Jenny's parents brought her back home, and she reconnected with her previous therapist. She quickly opened up about her intense sense of shame and humiliation. Her former ritualistic behaviors and phobias returned, with a fury. In addition to the OCD, Jenny was also diagnosed with panic disorder and acute stress reaction, a variation of PTSD.

Often patients with these diagnoses improve with treatment. But Jenny did not commit to therapy and refused to take medications. Weeks stretched into months, and she demonstrated little improvement. Soon Jenny settled into an uncomfortable routine, living in her childhood bedroom in her parents' home. She would not leave the house to find work. Her brother had moved on to a successful career in Chicago, and her friends from high school dwindled away.

Jenny's parents, Chris and Deborah, were torn by their daughter's plight and they sought professional help to work on their marriage. Two major issues served as the source of their recurrent conflict. The primary disagreement was financial. Chris believed that his daughter was not going to improve, and she would be dependent on the family for years. He felt that Jenny should apply for Supplemental Security Income (SSI). SSI is a federal program under the auspices of the Social Security Administration designed for low-income individuals who are permanently disabled by a medical or psychiatric illness, but who do not have a sufficient work history to qualify for Social Security disability insurance (SSDI). (The parents' income is not considered in the case of an adult.) Jenny herself offered no opinion about this issue.

But Deborah did. She objected vehemently to Chris's plan, and argued that seeking SSI would send the wrong message to Jenny. Deborah said, "If she gets SSI, then she will never work again and will not be motivated to try to get better." (In fact, individuals on SSI are encouraged to work, if they are able to do so.)

Chris countered that Jenny could work part-time and if she became well again she would no longer need the benefit. He also noted that with SSI, a person was automatically eligible for state Medicaid. Jenny could stay on his health insurance until age twenty-six, but what would happen when she was older? Her medications were expensive, and they would be covered by Medicaid.

The couple also disagreed about Jenny's relationship with her boyfriend, Michael. Michael did not have a high school diploma, and came from a broken family. Michael worked as a part-time baker for a doughnut shop, and earned very little. Nor did he seem interested in getting a better job.

Chris and Deborah had wanted more for their daughter than Michael, but Deborah knew that Jenny was not meeting other young men. Deborah was also grateful that Michael remained loyal to Jenny. But her husband was clear that he could not support the relationship. He believed Michael was a poor choice and said that Jenny was making an irreversibly bad decision. Chris said, "It's better that she be alone than to get pregnant and live a life of poverty." Deborah reminded Chris that Jenny was on birth control and was living in their home.

The conflict between the couple did not resolve easily, and Deborah and Chris received help from a family counselor for some time. In this process the family did come together and Jenny filed for SSI. After a long process and many forms, she was approved for SSI and Medicaid. The fear of a future financial burden was relieved.

Chris and Deborah determined that the decision about whether Jenny should date Michael (or anyone else) was not theirs to make. Jenny continued to see him. Although her parents found common ground from their therapy, Jenny did not seek help for her avoidant behavior. Chris and Deborah were disturbed by her inaction and they resolved that their next mission was to persuade Jenny to reengage in meaningful treatment for her anxiety disorder.

MOOD DISORDERS

The primary mood disorders are major depressive disorder and bipolar disorder. Major depressive disorder (MDD) affects about 7 percent of the population, and of this group, about 2 percent have a severe form of the disease. This disorder can occur at any age but the average age of onset is thirty-two, according to the National Institute of Mental Health (NIMH). About 2.6 percent of the adult population has bipolar disorder and most (83 percent) cases are classified as severe. With bipolar disorder, the average age of onset is twenty-five.

Major Depressive Disorder

Depressive episodes are characterized by periods of sad mood, a decreased interest in activities, and feelings of guilt, hopelessness, and worthlessness that last at least two weeks. Sleep and appetite disturbances may also occur, in which the individual sleeps excessively (or not enough) and eats too much (or not enough). Weight fluctuates and problems concentrating are noticeable. Suicidal thinking commonly occurs during periods of depression.

Antidepressants are used to treat major depression, and some of the antidepressants used for this illness have an iconic place in western culture. The serotonin reuptake inhibitors (SRIs) Prozac and Zoloft are nearly as well known in our society as Coke and Pepsi. These SRIs and other newer antidepressants have fewer severe side effects than older antidepressants such as imipramine, despiramine, and other drugs ending in "amine."

Depression is a common and debilitating problem that darkens the person's perceptions. In general, women are more likely to suffer from depression than men. Women with depression report feeling sad, excessively guilty, and worthless, while depressed men are more likely to suffer from insomnia and irritability and to misuse drugs and alcohol.

Depression may be triggered by external events, such as a loss of a job or the end of an important relationship. As frequently no new life problems are evident and the depression emerges for no apparent reason. There is evidence that biochemical alterations in the brain cause depression.

Depression tends to run in families and can be genetically transmitted. Major depressive disorder is distinguished from bipolar disorder by the absence of manic periods. Depression often accompanies other psychiatric disorders, such as anxiety disorders, ADHD, and chronic pain syndromes. About 40 percent of individuals with PTSD suffer from major depression. Dysthymia describes a chronic, low-level form of depression.

Antidepressant Medications
Prior to the 1990s, tricyclic antidepressants were used to treat most patients with depression, including drugs such as imipramine and desipramine. These drugs had more side effects than antidepressants developed since the late twentieth century. In the 1990s, the selective serotonin reuptake inhibitors (SSRIs) were dramatically introduced and became widely popular. SSRIs increase the level of circulating serotonin, thus easing depression. Examples of SSRIs include fluoxetine (Prozac), sertraline (Zoloft), paroxetine (Paxil), citalopram (Celexa), and escitalopram (Lexapro).

Several years later another class of antidepressants, the serotonin and norepinephrine reuptake inhibitors (SNRIs), were approved by the Food and Drug Administration (FDA) for depression treatment. SNRIs increase the blood levels of serotonin and norepinephrine, neurotransmitters that both regulate mood. Velafaxine (Effexor), duloxetine (Cymbalta), and desvenlafaxine (Pristiq) are prime examples.

Another commonly used antidepressant is bupropion (Wellbutrin). This medication affects the body's levels of the neurochemicals norepinephrine and dopamine. Vilazadone (Viibryd) is the most recent addition to the arsenal of available antidepressants. This medication was approved by the FDA in 2011.

Complications Associated with Treatment
Suicidal thoughts occur in up to 40 percent of patients suffering from depression. Usually once an individual responds to antidepressant treatment, these suicidal thoughts fade away. However, it has long been known

AMANDA: A CASE OF DEPRESSION

Amanda had suffered depressive episodes since childhood. In her early twenties, her symptoms subsided. During this period, Amanda worked in an electronics retail store and became a regional manager. She met Andre and they married and had two children. Their life together seemed to be on a positive course.

In the weeks following the birth of her second son, Amanda lapsed into a severe depression. She became tearful and reported profoundly sad feelings. Amanda lacked motivation to do anything. She slept twelve to fifteen hours per day and essentially neglected her young children.

Amanda's mother Linda reacted quickly to the crisis. She moved in with the family and began to manage the household. Andre worked sixty hours per week in his struggling restaurant, and both he and Amanda became highly dependent on Linda's help.

In the depths of her depression, Amanda spent most of her time in bed. She revealed to Linda that she hated being a mother and did not feel connected to her infant at all. She found darkness in all aspects of her life. She missed working and regretted her decision not to finish college. Amanda thought her husband was selfish and unsupportive and she asked her mother to contact a recently divorced friend for the name of her attorney. These revelations troubled Linda; she had never heard such global discontent from her daughter before.

Instead of helping Amanda find the attorney, Linda arranged for her daughter to consult with a psychiatrist. The doctor diagnosed Amanda with postpartum depression. An SSRI antidepressant medication was introduced initially, but it offered minimal benefit. After six weeks, a second medication was introduced to augment

that in the early stages of antidepressant treatment, the risk for suicide minimally increases, and for this reason, the FDA mandates that all antidepressants include a "black box" warning for consumers of this risk.

How could an antidepressant worsen a mood state? Experts speculate that antidepressants improve a patient's energy level days before their mood improves and thus, for a vulnerable period of time, the patient may have the energy to act on their self-harmful ideas. This phenomenon is more common in younger patients and the "black box" warning specifies that there is less concern for older patients.

the antidepressant and to everyone's relief, Amanda's mood greatly improved. As she recovered, her tenderness toward her children reappeared and talk of divorce subsided. Linda was able to return home and her daughter's family resumed their normal life.

Several months later, Amanda stopped taking her medications and within weeks, her depression and anxiety returned. As before she expressed her alienation from both her children and her husband, and again she talked of her desire to divorce. This time, Linda demanded that her daughter return to the psychiatrist immediately. Within seven days of restarting her medication, her anxiety and hostility diminished.

At that point, Linda insisted on meeting with Amanda and her psychiatrist. They discussed her two depressive episodes and identified that when Amanda became depressed, her thoughts became distorted. She viewed her life as bleak and became convinced that she had made many bad life decisions. The sense of worthlessness diminished as the depression lifted.

At the psychiatrist's direction Linda decided that part of her role as Amanda's mother was to encourage her daughter to stay in treatment. Andre remained angry at Amanda for her behavior. The doctor reminded Andre that depression was a chemical disorder that temporarily alters one's perspective. He emphasized that Amanda's hateful words and actions during her depression did not reflect her true feelings, and that their energy as a couple should be spent on maintaining her recovery rather than on dealing with irrelevant phantom issues.

It is important for parents of depressed adults to understand the distortions caused by depression. Do not overreact to the moment. Depressed individuals should be discouraged from quitting their job, breaking up relationships, or leaving their families. Life-altering decisions should not be made during this critical time.

It is important for the family to remember that antidepressant-induced suicidal behavior is an uncommon event, and the risk should be weighed against the many benefits that this class of medications delivers.

Bipolar Disorder

Bipolar disorder, sometimes called manic depression, is characterized by extreme mood swings. Periods of normal moods alternate with episodes of mania and depression. Bipolar depression is hard to distinguish from major depressive disorder, but experienced clinicians report that the symptoms are more severe. Suicidal behaviors may become particularly intense. (Read chapter 8 for more information about suicide.)

Mania is unique to bipolar disorder; it is a period of high energy that may last for several weeks. A manic patient reports racing thoughts and euphoria. He has an inflated sense of his abilities and exhibits impaired social judgment. Stories of extreme shopping sprees and impulsive sexual activity with unlikely partners are typical.

The higher the manic mood, the farther the person can fall down into depression. In the life course of a typical bipolar patient, depressed phases are more common than manic periods. Some patients alternate very quickly from mania to depression. Rapid cycling bipolar disorder is a variation that is less responsive to medications. Bipolar disorder may first appear in the late teens or early adulthood.

A person with severe bipolar disorder may also develop psychotic symptoms, such as hallucinations or delusions, particularly if she fails to take her medication. Psychosis can occur on both sides of the mood spectrum. A manic person may believe that the CIA has pegged him for a special assignment, while individuals with bipolar depression may develop the delusion that they have committed a crime. Neither of course is true, but these psychotic symptoms are dramatic and for this reason bipolar disorder is sometimes misdiagnosed as schizophrenia.

Individuals with bipolar disorder are at high risk for substance abuse and attention-deficit hyperactivity disorder (ADHD).

Treatment for Bipolar Disorder

Several different medications are known to help the symptoms of bipolar disorder. Lithium carbonate, derived from the natural element, was the standard medication for many decades. When it functions properly, lithium prevents the patient from falling into deep depression and protects him from reaching treacherous mania. However, lithium causes tremors and weight gain, and kidney and thyroid function needs to be carefully monitored with regular blood tests.

Because lithium is an imperfect drug, other mood stabilizers have been introduced for the treatment of bipolar disorder. These medications are

A CASE STUDY

Saul is a twenty-seven-year old medical student studying in Manhattan. He grew up in the Detroit area, and his parents, Henry and Rivka, remain there. They have four sons including Saul, all well educated and accomplished.

Saul became agitated during his third semester of medical school. At first, his parents attributed his behavior to a breakup with a long-term girlfriend. But over several weeks, Saul's irritability markedly accelerated. His sleep became erratic, and he lost weight. He stopped going to class and discarded his rent and monthly bills. His friends noted that Saul's alcohol consumption increased markedly.

Saul's brother Joshua became alarmed at his brother's frenetic pace and he contacted their father, who immediately flew to New York. Henry saw that his son was tired, irritable, and grandiose. Saul was convinced that he had a special relationship with God, and reported that God's voice was speaking to him.

Saul was loud and disruptive on the plane. It became clear that the air marshal was watching them both carefully and that Saul could have easily been thrown off the plane and arrested. Exasperated after the flight, Henry remembered: "The two-hour flight felt like a three-month pilgrimage. I sat on him the whole flight. It took my entire strength to contain him from going up to the cockpit."

Once home, Saul's erratic behavior continued undeterred. Henry and Rivka tried to keep him home, but he insisted on venturing out. Several weeks later, Saul was arrested for setting fire to a potted plant at the local library. He was taken to the hospital emergency room, where a merciful decision was made to consult a psychiatrist rather than the local police.

During his psychiatric hospitalization, Saul was diagnosed with bipolar disorder. A treatment plan, including medications and therapy, was established. Henry and Rivka agreed with the plan, but Saul was not convinced. Once discharged, he rarely took his medications and skipped most of the appointments with the therapist. This unproductive routine went on for several more weeks.

During this period, Henry and Rivka were mortified at their son's decreased need for sleep, his overspending, and his heavy alcohol use. He was also sexually inappropriate and continued to have auditory hallucinations. The new Saul was very different than the old one and his parents sorely missed the original version. Normally very dignified people, Henry and Rivka grew to believe that

Saul's manic behavior would never resolve. They cursed at their son, fought with each other, and were nasty to the doctor's office staff.

It did not take long for the treatment team to conclude that Saul was a very difficult patient because his parents were so off-putting, and to assume that Saul had patterned himself after the bad behavior of his awful mother and father. Despite the rocky relationship with the family, the team stayed focused on Saul's treatment.

Then, after months of chaos, Saul began to take his medications. Within a week, his mood stabilized and his grandiosity diminished. Three weeks later, the original Saul reemerged. He was pleasant, cooperative, bright, and compassionate. It was hard to imagine that he had been such a different character several months earlier. His parents reconstituted as well. As Saul stabilized, they returned to their civil and polite selves.

Saul soon returned to school in New York. He now checks in four times yearly. He no longer drinks alcohol and is on mood-stabilizing medications. There have been no further manic or depressive periods.

Saul's case highlights several issues for the parents of bipolar adult children. Most importantly, despite a period of severe mania, Saul did get better. Accurate diagnosis and tenacious treatment, while not immediate, did eventually help him.

Secondly, Saul's rapid decline placed enormous pressure on his family and it warped his parent's relationships. When Saul was ill, Henry and Rivka became negative and argumentative. Out of fear, they became over-involved in their son's life and alienated him and his treatment team. Once Saul rebounded, the tension in these relationships diminished.

When caring parents witness their children spiral out of control, desperation often sets in. If they could, parents would try to spin on their nose if it would help their children. When there is recovery, normal family relationships usually do return. It is very easy for friends and professionals to blame adult parents for their adult child's mental illness. In most cases, however, the child is ill because he has a biological condition, not because of any parental failing. The illness should be attacked and the temptation to blame parents should be resisted.

less effective than lithium but they are better tolerated. Divalproex sodium (Depakote), gabapentin (Neurontin), topiramate (Topamax), oxcarbamazepine (Trileptal), and lamotrigine (Lamictal) were first used by neurologists for seizure disorders.

Some atypical antipsychotic medications have been used to treat bipolar disorder, such as olanzapine (Zyprexa), aripiprazole (Abilify), quetiapine (Seroquel), risperidone (Risperdal), and asenapine (Saphris). Antidepressants are commonly used to treat the depressive episodes of bipolar disorder.

If bipolar disorder is treated, your child's life may be indistinguishable from any other adult's. However, if the condition is not properly diagnosed and treated or she stops taking her medication, parents may feel like they are trapped in the middle of a maelstrom.

ARE SOME MENTAL DISORDERS CAUSED BY SPECIFIC GENETIC ABNORMALITIES?

Cutting edge research on the genetic components of psychiatric illnesses is starting to uncover the particular genes that may be implicated in severe psychiatric disorders. The results of a study published in *Lancet* in 2013 offer evidence that specific genes are associated with major mental illness. In this study, 33,332 cases of people with autism, ADHD, bipolar disorder, depression, and schizophrenia were compared to 27,888 individuals in a control group. The researchers found specific genetic locations for bipolar disorder and schizophrenia and also linked the genetics of all five psychiatric disorders.

This research supports previous research that demonstrated a genetic underpinning to mental illness. The emerging field of psychogenetics one day may lead to more effective ways to treat psychiatric disorders, although these solutions are years away.

Key Symptoms of and Treatments for Selected Psychiatric Disorders

Disease	Key Symptoms	Medications	Therapy
Antisocial personality disorder	Defined by behavior, such as committing criminal acts and not considering the feelings or beliefs of others. The person may lie, cheat, steal, or do whatever he feels will achieve his goals. Yet there is no remorse. Sometimes the individual is referred to as a sociopath.	No specific medications are used.	These patients usually do not identify that they have a problem and rarely seek psychotherapy or take treatment seriously.
Anxiety disorder: generalized anxiety disorder	Extreme worry over real or imagined problems to the point that the person can't sleep and can't concentrate on daily life issues.	SSRI and SNRI antidepressants over the long term	Cognitive behavioral therapy and supportive therapy
Anxiety disorder: obsessive-compulsive disorder	Constant thinking about performing rituals such as excessive handwashing, counting things, and repetitive checking for things, such as whether the door is locked.	SSRI antidepressants, especially sertraline (Zoloft), paroxetine (Paxil), and fluoxetine (Prozac)	Cognitive behavioral therapy and supportive therapy; exposure therapy
Anxiety disorder: panic disorder	Racing and pounding heart and severe sweating. Person may feel like she is having a heart attack.	Benzodiazepines such as lorazepam (Ativan) and alprazolam (Xanax) can be used in the short run. Also antidepressants.	Cognitive behavioral therapy and supportive therapy
Anxiety disorder: PTSD	Flashbacks; easy startling (hyperarousability); nightmares	Antidepressants such as sertraline (Zoloft) or paroxetine (Paxil)	Cognitive behavioral therapy, exposure and supportive therapy

Disease	Key Symptoms	Medications	Therapy
ADHD	Extreme impulsivity; inability to concentrate; blurting out comments that are inappropriate. Severe ADHD may sometimes be misdiagnosed as bipolar disorder. However, the cyclical nature of mania/depression is not present with severe ADHD. Only an experienced psychiatrist can diagnose this disorder.	Stimulants such as long-acting methylphenidate (Concerta, Focalin) or long-acting amphetamine (Adderall XR, Vyvanse) and non-stimulants, such as guanfacine (Intuniv), clonidine extended release (Kapvay), or atomoxetine (Strattera)	ADHD coaching and supportive therapy. Family therapy can be useful.
Mild autism spectrum disorder (formerly known as Asperger's syndrome)	Severe social problems; tics that may be misdiagnosed as Tourette's syndrome.	No specific medications are indicated. Atypical antispychotics, such as risperidone (Risperdal) are used for behavioral disruption in children with mild ASD. Underlying mood disorders and ADHD are treated with antidepressants, mood-stabilizing agents, and stimulant medications.	Supportive individual therapy. Group therapy focused on life skills.
Bipolar disorder	Mania alternating with depression. Manic acts may include hypersexuality and excessive spending. Depressive acts may include changes in sleeping (too much or not enough) and changes in eating (too much or not enough). The individual may become suicidal in the depressive state.	Lithium; mood stabilizers such as divalproex sodium (Depakote) or anticonvulsants such as gabapentin (Neurontin), topiramate (Topamax), oxcarbazepine (Trileptal), and lamotrigine (Lamictal). May also be treated with atypical antipsychotics, such as olanzapine (Zyprexa), aripiprazole (Abilify), quetiapine (Seroquel), risperidone (Risperdal), and asenapine (Saphris).	Supportive therapy. Group therapy.

Disease	Key Symptoms	Medications	Therapy
Borderline personality disorder	Reckless and impulsive behavior. May be difficult to distinguish from bipolar disorder.	There is no medication that is specifically approved by the Food and Drug Administration (FDA) for borderline personality disorder. Concurrent mood disorders or ADHD should be treated.	Dialectical behavioral therapy
Major depression	Loss of interest in former activities that the person enjoyed, changes in sleeping (too much or not enough), changes in eating (too much or not enough). Headaches or digestive problems that do not improve with treatment. Person may become suicidal.	Many different antidepressants; atypical antipsychotics for treatment-resistant depression	Individual therapy, cognitive behavioral therapy
Intermittent explosive disorder (IED)	Rage attacks—usually unprovoked	Various medications are used with inconsistent results. Anti-seizure medications, antidepressants, antipsychotics, and psychostimulants may all play a role.	Psychotherapy may help. Brain imaging may be helpful.
Schizophrenia	Psychotic symptoms such as auditory hallucinations and delusions; confused speech, flat affect (no emotion)	Atypical antipsychotics such as olanzapine (Zyprexa), aripiprazole (Abilify), quetiapine (Seroquel XR), risperidone (Risperdal) and ziprasidone (Geodon); older typical antipsychotics	Supportive therapy. Group therapy focused on life and social skills.

SCHIZOPHRENIA

According to the National Institute of Mental Health (NIMH), about 1 percent of all people in the United States have chronic paranoid schizophrenia. The causes of schizophrenia are unknown but have been studied for years. Past generations felt that schizophrenia was caused by cold mothers, but this theory has been abandoned. The current belief is schizophrenia is largely inherited although exposure to an environmental toxin or a virus is also a possibility. Schizophrenia usually starts in late adolescence or the twenties and has a devastating impact on the individual and his family. Schizophrenia is one of the most highly researched fields in psychiatry.

What Are the Symptoms of Schizophrenia?

Schizophrenia is characterized by psychosis, or an inability to differentiate reality from misperceptions. Common symptoms include auditory hallucinations, internal voices that offer running commentary and delusions, fixed false beliefs that people are out to "get" you, or the belief that secret messages are embedded in movies or on television.

Schizophrenic symptoms are generally categorized as either positive or negative. Positive symptoms are not "good," nor are negative symptoms "bad." Instead, positive symptoms may cause externalizing behaviors, while negative behaviors are internalizing. Positive symptoms include delusions, hallucinations, and thought disorders, such as a fear that someone is plotting against you.

Positive symptoms may lead to individuals acting out. For example, if your adult child has a delusion that someone is threatening him, he might respond to the threat with aggressive behavior. When these symptoms are present, the behavior of a person with schizophrenia is more unpredictable.

Negative symptoms of the schizophrenic experience describe a blunted emotional life and an inability to form social relationships. They are unable to plan and pursue pleasurable activities. The person with schizophrenia may speak very little and struggle with personal hygiene and everyday tasks. Negative symptoms are responsible for a withdrawal from life.

Medications and Other Treatments for Schizophrenia

Schizophrenia is treated with antipsychotic medications, and patients can feel and function much better after a short exposure. For years various neuroleptics were the mainstay of treatment, including thioridazine (Mellaril) and haloperidol (Haldol). Atypical antipsychotics were introduced twenty years ago and have become standard treatment. This class includes aripiprazole (Abilify), paliperidone (Invega), olanzapine (Zyprexa), risperidone (Risperdal), quetiapine (Seroquel), and ziprasidone (Geodon).

To varying degrees, all of these medications have side effects. Significant weight gain is common and this increases the risk for type 2 diabetes. Patients may also develop movement disorders, muscle tightness, internal restlessness, or involuntary facial movements, although these treatment complications are more commonly associated with older antipsychotics such as haloperidol and thioridazine rather than with the newer atypical antipsychotic medications like aripiprazole (Abilify).

Beyond treatment with medications, an effective treatment plan for a person with schizophrenia includes interpersonal counseling as well as providing education about the disease, and practical guidance about getting and maintaining jobs, relationships, and housing.

Problems with Medication Compliance

Individuals with schizophrenia struggle with medication compliance. Patients stop taking their medication because of side effects. Most deeply dislike the weight gain, excessive salivation, and the drowsiness that comes with antipsychotic medications. Schizophrenic patients may develop a false belief that they have already been "cured." For patients who cannot maintain a daily schedule of oral medications, long-acting injectable forms are available for administration every two to four weeks.

The Risk for Violence

Most people with schizophrenia are not usually dangerous. Their behavior is more unpredictable if they are also abusing alcohol or other drugs. Marijuana and stimulants can worsen schizophrenic symptoms. Suicide is a pressing concern, and an estimated 10 percent of young males with schizophrenia die from suicide, according to the National Institute of Mental Health (NIMH).

JASON: BREAKING BAD

Jason was a popular high school student who was selected as captain of his lacrosse team. His parents, Myrna and Jack, were rightfully proud of him, and after graduation they sent Jason to a small college. His first semester went well, although a few too many weekends were spent partying. Halfway through his second semester, Jack and Myrna learned that his grades were poor. Jason also disclosed to his parents that he was smoking marijuana daily.

Jason's performance continued to deteriorate. His parents questioned him, and Jason disclosed that since members of his fraternity were working against him, he had to drop out and live elsewhere. At first, his parents were supportive; they were not surprised that Jason had taken a dislike to Greek life. It became clear, however, that Jason's problems were greater than fraternity politics.

The next weekend Jason came home, exasperated that his roommate was working with the university administration to video monitor him. By the end of the semester, Jason's parents had received word from his friends that he was walking around campus talking to himself. One Saturday night, intoxicated and disheveled, Jason threw a rock through a library window.

After a night in jail, Jason was seen by a psychiatrist, who gave a diagnosis of substance abuse and psychosis. The doctor also stated that since drugs and alcohol could cause paranoid behavior, Jason would need to get clean and sober. Jason was admitted into a psychiatric hospital and for three weeks, he was physically unable to access alcohol or marijuana. Despite this forced sobriety, Jason's psychotic delusions persisted. At a family meeting, the treatment team informed Jason and his family that he had schizophrenia.

Jason's case typifies a schizophrenic break. Symptoms emerge out of the blue, often early in college or during military basic training. The first signs may present during periods of excessive substance use. In fact, one misconception is that schizophrenia is caused by substances. Instead, the person with schizophrenia turns to substances to try to block out their psychotic symptoms. If the psychosis continues in the absence of alcohol and other drugs, then a diagnosis of schizophrenia is usually confirmed.

Jack and Myrna had to adjust to living with a son with schizophrenia. Jason's hallucinations were very real for him, and his parents soon learned that they could not convince him that the internal voices were symptoms of an illness. His paranoid convictions were deeply held and his behavior was erratic. In the first two years following his diagnosis, Myrna and Jack had to involuntarily hospitalize Jason twice.

Over time, Jason's positive symptoms, hallucinations and delusions, were muted by antipsychotic medications. His negative symptoms became the primary problem. He was unable to return to school and was poorly motivated to hold down basic jobs. Every day his parents had to push him to keep showered and shaved.

At the same time that they were doing battle with Jason's symptoms, Jack and Myrna had to cope with their lost hopes. Australian psychologist Meg Richardson reviewed studies on parental reactions to their adult child's mental illness, and found that most parents of mentally ill children experience deep and ongoing sorrow. Relationships throughout the family become tense and compromised.

For parents of adult children with schizophrenia, the grief gets worse. Most parents do not understand the full implications of the illness when it is first diagnosed. They learn that medications and other treatments do help, but soon realize that full recovery is unlikely. One study reports that parents of an adult child with schizophrenia experience grief at levels that rival or exceed the grief of parents whose child has died. Very few of these parents get psychological help.

Jack and Myrna needed help. They became physically and emotionally exhausted by their son's illness. The financial burden of caring for him became overwhelming. They were gratified that the newly enacted Affordable Care Act allowed them to keep Jason on their private health insurance until his twenty-sixth birthday. On his bittersweet twenty-seventh birthday, Jason received a smartphone from Jack and Myrna, and a Medicaid card for public insurance from the state of Michigan. His first Social Security disability check arrived shortly thereafter.

OTHER SERIOUS PSYCHIATRIC DISORDERS

Many people with psychiatric disorders can differentiate reality from unreality, but their psychiatric problems make it very difficult for them to function effectively. There are many such disorders, but the rest of this chapter concentrates on attention-deficit hyperactivity disorder (ADHD) and the antisocial and borderline personality disorders, as well as taking a brief look at intermittent explosive disorder (IED). We also offer an overview of mild autism spectrum disorder, formely known as Asperger's syndrome.

Adult Attention-Deficit Hyperactivity Disorder (ADHD)

Current estimates are that ADHD is present in about 4.4 percent of the adult population in the United States. The diagnostic criteria for adults with this condition will soon be updated and will likely reflect a prevalence rate that is nearly equal to the percentage found in children (7 to 9 percent of the population). ADHD usually appears in childhood, and contrary to popular belief, ADHD usually continues into adulthood in the majority of cases.

ADHD is characterized by excessive hyperactivity and impulsivity and/ or inattention. It causes impairment in daily functioning. Not all individuals with ADHD have all these symptoms in equal parts; usually one or two of the symptoms predominate. For example, hyperactivity and impulsivity travel together, and individuals with these symptoms struggle to sit through school classes or important meetings. They act without thinking and their actions can rub others in the wrong way.

Other individuals with ADHD seem lost in a daydream much of the time. The inattentive person with ADHD may find that she is underemployed because she has trouble focusing on learning new tasks. She may be highly disorganized, an erratic driver, and may struggle to get tasks done. Inattentive individuals develop a reputation for being undependable, a moniker that is hard to shake because it is often accurate.

ADHD and Problem Behaviors

ADHD is an invisible disorder that is often trivialized in the media. Parents of children with ADHD understand their children's struggle and now researchers are starting to capture the magnitude of the disorder. Several years ago, Timothy Wilens and his colleagues at the Massachusetts General Hospital identified that adolescents with ADHD had an elevated risk for developing substance disorders.

Other researchers found that when ADHD adults were compared to non-ADHD adults, they had a lower educational achievement, a lower yearly income, more divorces, and more criminal arrests. Roughly 30 to 40 percent of long-serving criminals have ADHD.

Barbaresi and colleagues combed through the medical records of 367 individuals who were diagnosed with ADHD in childhood, reporting their results in *Pediatrics* in 2013. They found that compared to a large comparison group, adults with ADHD were more likely to have a substance abuse disorder, anxiety disorder, or depression. Most disturbingly they had higher rates of suicide.

Treatment for ADHD

There is increasing evidence that treatment for ADHD helps over the life span. A large Swedish study tracked 25,000 ADHD subjects over four years. The researchers found that men with ADHD who took approved ADHD medications showed nearly a one-third reduction in their crime rate (32 percent). ADHD women who complied with treatment had a 41 percent decrease in crime. This finding did not apply to other psychiatric medications; the researchers found no crime reduction rate among the subjects who had taken an SSRI antidepressant.

The dilemma of parents reading this book is where to draw the boundary between themselves and their troubled adult child. Finding that perfect place where helping your child does not interfere with his free will is hard, and parents will need to find their own comfort zone. However, on one point we are adamant. If your child has treatable psychiatric conditions, particularly ADHD, then making every provision for him to obtain medication treatment will fundamentally improve his chance of success. Ensuring medication treatment is different from making your child's decisions for him or living her life for her. Rather it helps them avoid the pitfalls of ADHD and allows them a fighting chance at happiness.

Explosive Anger: Intermittent Explosive Disorder (IED)

A person who has periodic uncontrollable rages may have *intermittent explosive disorder*. IED is categorized with other impulse control disorders such as pathological gambling, trichotillomania (compulsive hair pulling), pyromania (compulsive fire-setting), and kleptomania (stealing objects that one does not want or need). One common example of IED behavior is "road rage." These individuals become enraged by other drivers, even if the offense was unintentional. They retaliate in a manner that is completely disproportionate to the real or perceived insult. It is not uncommon for the enraged person with IED to follow the other driver, verbally berate him, and sometimes threaten assault. Police departments and judges generally do not tolerate this behavior.

Prior to an explosion, the person with IED may experience a pattern of hyperarousal, anxiety, and racing thoughts, as well as excessive energy and the compulsion to defend themselves from real or imagined insults. Explosive individuals lose all rational control when in a rage state.

Some clinicians believe that compulsive shoplifting is another manifestation of IED. Shoplifters are usually female. They steal not so much for the economic benefit but for the thrill. Compulsive shoplifters describe many of the same aspects of the arousal pattern seen with IED. They are highly energized when planning and executing their action, but in the end, they find it to be anticlimactic.

Family members of individuals with IED are never at ease. Any disruption that their child encounters, such as waiting in line or being treated rudely in a chance encounter, can provoke an exaggerated response. Families live in a constant state of fear that self-destruction lies around the corner. Families are forced into a stance of passivity, wary that anything they say or do could provoke an extreme reaction.

Waiting for the Explosion

Many families cannot maintain their composure. Brenda's adult son Derek had severe IED and she could not remember the number of times that she had repaired her home after he had put a fist through the drywall. Brenda said, "Derek's worst explosions have occurred at the bar, but my husband also aggravates the situation at home. He comments about Derek's every movement. Many times, my husband could just walk away, but instead, he always feels a need to teach a life lesson. They have so many angry exchanges about Derek being late or forgetful, and Derek can't tolerate the pestering. His outbursts happen all the time, but my husband always seems surprised that Derek has not outgrown them. My husband blames me for being permissive and allowing Derek to act this way and I suppose I blame my husband for being pigheaded. We are always fighting about Derek."

IED Treatment

There are no approved FDA treatments for IED. In fact, psychiatric symptoms that are intermittent are sometimes harder to treat than symptoms that appear on a daily basis. IED has to be distinguished from other psychiatric conditions such as bipolar disorder, ADHD, and antisocial personality disorder, but medications that address these conditions also appear to decrease the frequency and intensity of the periodic outbursts.

Family members may benefit considerably from counseling. For example, Derek's family would have benefited from a strategy designed to decrease unnecessary provocations. A family therapist would explain to Derek that his outbursts are highly disruptive to his family and that he needs to take responsibility for his actions. At the same time the therapist can instruct a "less is more" strategy: It is counterproductive to criticize Derek's every move or to have the same family argument night after night. The fact that Derek does not have complete control over his behavior should also be acknowledged. Family therapy allows a safe haven for spouses to be reminded that their frustration is about their child and not each other.

Personality Disorders

Individuals with personality disorders have enduring behaviors that interfere with functioning and complicate interpersonal relationships. This small section will discuss the antisocial and borderline personality disorders and their impact on families.

Antisocial Personality Disorder

Antisocial personality disorder (ASPD) is defined by the person's behavior, rather than by how he feels inside. Although ASPD can only be diagnosed in individuals older than eighteen, their antisocial features do not suddenly emerge on their eighteenth birthday. Most have a childhood history of behavioral disturbances, and adults with ASPD likely demonstrated oppositional defiant disorder (ODD) or conduct disorder (CD) earlier in life. Men are more likely than women to have ASPD.

The person with ASPD does not respect authority and as a result pushes the limits of all rules and laws. Some adults with ASPD are violent and they are also overrepresented in prison populations. Adults with ASPD may also be sociopaths, or individuals who have no empathy for their victims. Sociopaths can be hard to detect; they often demonstrate normal facial expressions and gestures, but this is pure theater. Internally they do not possess or process genuine emotions. Individuals with ASPD easily manipulate others, lie freely, and steal without hesitation. Attempts may be made to treat the personality disorder with therapy. ASPD patients rarely take these efforts seriously and unless forced during incarceration, they usually do not follow through with treatment.

An individual with ASPD has many victims, but few who suffer more than his own family. Parents with children who have ASPD often witness their children doing unspeakable things. The family of an ASPD child is not responsible for his misdeeds, but they may spend a lifetime trying to right the many wrongs. ASPD adult children have high rates of being adopted. This raises a question: Is ASPD genetically predetermined, or does it result from the trauma of being separated at an early age from a biological parent? Both biological and adoptive families of adult children with ASPD benefit from counseling, not because there is much to be done, but because it is therapeutic to talk about the human tornado that revisits their home.

Borderline Personality Disorder

Borderline personality disorder is characterized by reckless and impulsive behavior, difficulty managing one's thoughts and emotions, and unstable relationships with others. Women are more commonly diagnosed with BPD than men, and an estimated 1.6 percent of the American population has this condition.

In some cases, the person with borderline personality disorder may experience brief episodes of psychosis or of dissociation. Dissociation is an eerie sensation that a person is operating outside and beyond the body. During these dissociative states, borderline patients are prone to cut their wrists, bang their heads, or burn themselves. They also "live on the edge," and may migrate to dangerous behaviors. They are likely to abuse substances, participate in unsafe sex, binge and purge, and shoplift.

Individuals with borderline personality disorder are more likely than others to have been victims of childhood abuse, but they may feel ashamed by their past experience. Severe mood swings reflect their emotional pain. Their threats of self-harm represent both a lost sense of self-control and a desire to manipulate others.

Patients with borderline personality disorder explain that cutting themselves makes them feel "alive." Self-injury temporarily reduces their internal tension and fulfills a need for self-punishment. These acts are usually not lethal, but about 5 percent of borderline patients will eventually commit suicide.

Women with BPD are often notoriously poor mothers, and they may hostilely control their children or ignore them altogether. Such parenting may lead to terrible outcomes for their children. It's a case of a victim creating a new victim.

Individuals with borderline personality disorder sometimes idealize their family members, while at other times, they demonize them. One day, you are the most wonderful person in the world, and then a few days later, you are evil. This unpredictable behavior is very confusing to the parents of adult children with BPD.

If the person with borderline personality disorder is willing to be treated, which is not always the case, then cognitive-behavioral therapy techniques are often recommended. Cognitive-behavioral therapy (CBT) teaches individuals to challenge their own internal automatic and irrational thoughts and to replace them with more rational thoughts. For example, the CBT therapist will help the patient replace the assertion that "My parents are evil!" with the more accurate concept that, "My parents are ordinary people who do their best."

Dialectical behavior therapy (DBT) uses similar principles and is applied in individual and group therapy with borderline patients. This type of therapy teaches the person to be mindfully aware of what is going on at specific given times so that she can better control her extreme emotions. It also helps to reduce the incidences of self-destructive behaviors.

There are no FDA-approved drugs that are specifically targeted to treat borderline personality disorder, but up to 85 percent of those with borderline personality disorder have other treatable disorders, such as anxiety, depression, or ADHD. These conditions should be treated with the appropriate medications.

MILD AUTISM SPECTRUM DISORDER

Children and adults with mild autism spectrum disorder (formerly known as Asperger's syndrome) are on the continuum of autism spectrum disorders (ASDs). These overlapping disorders have been described for years but scantily researched. We know that they can bring considerable heartbreak to their families.

Mild ASD is characterized by an awkward interpersonal style and social withdrawal. Individuals with this disorder are inept at reading body language and nonverbal communication. They are often smart and may cultivate an intense interest in limited topics. For example, they can become top experts in coins, comic books, or carburetors and may master endless information on these topics.

The problem is that individuals with mild ASD usually have few friends to share their interests. They are physically clumsy and often have distinctive physical features that distinguish them from the group. As children they are likely to be ostracized and bullied by their peers and their social isolation can last a lifetime. Parents of children with mild ASD witness their child's social rejection from their earliest interaction. Adults with this disorder have little recourse but to endure the pain quietly.

Or do they? The entire country was heartbroken in the aftermath of the 2012 massacre of twenty elementary school children and six of their teachers in Newtown, Connecticut. Adam Lanza, the young man who masterminded the massacre, had mild autism spectrum disorder. He had few friends and his mother apparently devoted her adult life to placating her troubled adult child. In this effort, she made a terrible mistake by introducing him to firearms. She was his first victim.

Clinicians are increasingly concerned about the psychological consequences of longstanding social rejection. Adults with mild ASD crave friendship, and they need social acceptance and a sexual connection. To have these needs denied, often cruelly, must leave lasting wounds. We will never know if these factors contributed to the rage that drove Adam Lanza's evil actions.

In the aftermath of this episode, mental health professionals were deluged with calls from parents of adult children with mild ASD, asking if their child had the same potential for extreme violence. Wise clinicians were able to reassure callers that most adults with this disorder are not violent, but the mental health community was unable to give complete reassurance. The incident at Newtown focuses us to try to more fully understand the fate of folks with these disorders.

SUPPORT GROUPS FOR ADULT CHILDREN AND THEIR PARENTS

The National Alliance for Mental Illness (NAMI) is a nationwide organization in the United States with local chapters. NAMI provides information and support to the families of the mentally ill as well as to the mentally ill themselves. There are also often local support groups for both family members and mentally ill individuals. Talking with others who are experiencing similar problems can be extremely helpful for many people who previously had felt alone with their struggles.

KEY POINTS IN THIS CHAPTER

- Many psychiatric problems cause stress and tension among parents of adult children.

- Adult children with schizophrenia, bipolar disorder, anxiety disorders, and other mental illnesses actively need treatment.

- Medications that are specifically targeted to the diagnosed illness may help considerably.

- Problems with medication compliance (taking medication as ordered by a physician) are common among people with mental disorders.

The next chapter covers a very serious and painful topic: suicide.

CHAPTER 8
SUICIDAL BEHAVIOR

It was a Tuesday morning and Marie was checking her e-mail. She knew her twenty-four-year-old son Michael was struggling hard with daily life. He was a bright, anxious, and socially withdrawn young man. After high school graduation, Michael chose to attend college far from his hometown. Overwhelmed at this large school, Michael never quite fit in. After graduation, a scholarship to a prestigious master's program boosted his confidence—for a while. Then he met a girl, his first real relationship, and Michael felt everything was progressing well. But within a month, his girlfriend started postponing dates and failing to return his texts. Michael felt blindsided and was distraught about the breakup.

As Marie read a new e-mail from Michael, she was shocked. It said, "Mom—I can't take this anymore. I can't stay happy and I hate being lonely. I can't go on." Before she read the entire note, Marie called Michael in a panic. As the phone rang and rang, then going to voice mail, she wondered, "Can I reach him in time?"

Another high stakes drama was playing out in the same city, where Nancy had received a call from Michelle, her son Cole's wife. Cole was angry and upset and yet again was threatening suicide. "You deal with him," Michelle had said. "I can't handle it anymore."

Nancy had adopted Cole, now twenty-eight, as an infant. Cole was provided with lots of love, but never seemed to find his place in life. Cole had ADHD and a severe learning disability and school was a negative experience for him. As a teenager, he found validation working in his father's scrap metal business. Around that time, Cole also told his parents he was gay, but never was willing to discuss the issue further. His father's sudden death left him without a confidant or a protected place to work

During the next few years, Cole knocked about, took a few courses, and had a few jobs. When he was twenty-six, Cole suddenly married Michelle, a thirty-four-year-old mother of two teenage children. Nancy wondered but didn't ask Cole about his earlier declaration of being gay. Nancy was supportive of her son's new family, and gratified Cole had found someone important in his life. But Nancy's enthusi-

140

asm had waned in the past year when she began receiving desperate phone calls from Michelle. Cole was constantly provoking fights with Michelle and her sons. Worse, every few weeks he threatened to harm himself, and Nancy and Michelle together had taken him to the emergency room twice. After this newest call from Michelle, Nancy desperately wondered what to do. Should she initiate another psychiatric hospitalization? Was Cole's threat of suicide even real?

When you are parenting your child as a baby, young child, or even during the tumultuous teenage years, you could never imagine that your child could become so very unhappy as an adult that he would attempt and perhaps succeed at ending his life. In those more innocent times, it is inconceivable that he might reject the most precious gift you have given him—his life. Yet all too often, parents of troubled adult children grapple with this unthinkable possibility.

The questions that Marie and Nancy asked themselves at the beginning of this chapter are difficult issues for even experienced mental health professionals to answer. The risk of suicide is vivid for those in the midst of emotional turmoil, and many times parents are forced to make life and death decisions for their children in crisis. In the aftermath, parents must wrestle with the emotional impact of having a child who has so little self-regard that he would attempt to end his own life. The consequences of a completed suicide are far greater.

Suicide attempts compel parents to realize that they have only finite control over their adult children. They realize that the forces of self-destruction that lie within a suicidal adult are powerful and often unsuppressible. These forces are often driven by strong elements such as mental illness, substance abuse, rage, and humiliation. Of course, not all suicidal behaviors are driven by the same elements, most suicide attempts do not end in death, and every event requires a separate analysis.

Michael and Cole from the beginning of this chapter had different outcomes, which are described later in this chapter. They represent examples of two families facing their son's self-imposed mortal danger. This chapter covers the complexities of suicidal behaviors and the key risk factors for suicide. It also offers suggestions for ways parents can intervene when their child is at the brink. The chapter ends with a discussion of the impossible task of coping with a child's death that has occurred at his own hands.

DEFINING THE PROBLEM

About 38,000 Americans ended their lives through suicide in 2010, according to the Centers for Disease Control and Prevention (CDC), and suicide is the tenth leading cause of death in the United States. In addition, an estimated one million people reported making a suicide attempt within the past year, and nearly four times that percentage thought about committing suicide. The CDC reports that for every one suicide, there are an attempted twenty-five suicides.

Men have a significantly greater risk of dying from suicide than women, and men represent nearly 80 percent of all completed suicides in the United States. Men and women also differ with respect to the means that they use to commit suicide; the CDC reports that 56 percent of men who commit suicide use firearms, while suicidal women are most likely to poison themselves by overdose.

In considering the age of a person and the risk for suicide, the CDC reports that young adults ages eighteen to twenty-nine years have a significantly higher rate of suicidal thoughts, suicide planning, and suicide attempts when compared to adults thirty years and older. Ironically, those individuals who are in what should be the sweetest part of their lives are thinking about ending their journey. The presence of mental illness and substance abuse often accounts for these alarming figures.

CALIFORNIA (UNHAPPY) DREAMING

Some Californians are very unhappy. The UCLA Center for Health Policy Research issued an extensive study of suicide in California in 2012. The researchers estimated that in 2009, more than a half million Californian adults seriously considered suicide and 60,000 had made a suicidal attempt in the past month. This report noted that 3,675 Californians died from suicide in 2009.

TYPES OF SUICIDAL BEHAVIORS

Mental health professionals designate different types of self-harmful behaviors. The least lethal form of suicidal behavior is referred to as passive suicidal thoughts, followed in terms of risk by those with active suicidal thoughts, then those who have made suicidal gestures or unsuccessful attempts. The completed suicide is the most severe form of suicidal behavior.

Passive Suicidal Thoughts

These depressed patients relate that they have thoughts about "not waking up" or "just not being here." When pressed, they deny that they have an active suicide plan and dismiss the possibility that they would ever harm themselves. These are unsettling thoughts to hear, but they usually do not represent an imminent risk.

Active Suicidal Thoughts

Individuals with active suicidal thoughts do ponder their own deaths, even if they never act on these thoughts. A person with active suicidal thoughts is burdened by disturbing images and thoughts, and may make statements such as, "I drive by the railroad every morning and think about driving my car on to the tracks and staying there, but I have never done it."

Surprisingly, for many people these recurrent troubling thoughts never go any further. However, concern grows if and when these individuals develop an actual plan for their own self-destruction, such as, "I plan to hang myself after my parents leave for work next week." If such thoughts are expressed to relatives or friends, they demand serious attention.

Suicidal Gestures, Unsuccessful Attempts, and Completed Suicides

Suicidal thoughts that evolve into behaviors are of great concern. Suicidal acts are subdivided into gestures, unsuccessful attempts, or completed suicides, in which the person self-harms and dies.

Suicidal gestures include such acts as swallowing three or four sleeping pills or superficially cutting one's wrists. Hospital emergency rooms are filled with patients with these mild injuries, and the generally accepted belief is that these are impulsive acts rather than well-planned acts. These individuals need psychological help but do not plan to die from their injuries.

Every hospital has what some refer to as "frequent flyers," or notorious patients who make repeated suicidal gestures. These patients carry the scars of healed lacerations, and their medical charts are stuffed with information on past medical encounters. Each episode is disruptive to the family and costly for the hospital. Suicidal gestures are often considered manipulative or attention-seeking behaviors intended to provoke a sympathetic response. As the gestures become more frequent, sympathy inevitably morphs into resentment. However, it is a serious mistake for anyone to turn a cold shoulder to this behavior. Suicidal gestures always represent underlying emotional distress. Even the most benign self-harmful gestures can go wrong and result in an unintentional death.

Suicidal behaviors that do not end in death have the ironic designation of an "unsuccessful attempt." These patients intend to die from their actions, but instead they survived because they miscalculated the number of pills needed to die or some heroic medical effort was made to save them. Survivors are at great risk for subsequent attempts. But the outcome is not always bad.

Eileen was a fifty-five-year-old patient with bipolar disorder who survived a massive drug overdose years earlier. In Hebrew, the number eighteen is called *chai*, and it also represents life. I was surprised one day to find an invitation to Eileen's "Chai party." The invitation read: "On this eighteenth anniversary of my survival, I wish to celebrate my life."

With a completed suicide, the attempt results in death. Death is delivered by a gunshot wound, overdose, a hanging, or other means. For a doctor, a completed suicide represents the worst possible outcome (short of homicide-suicide). For the surviving family, suicide marks the beginning of the darkest chapter imaginable. The death of a child from suicide places parents in the black hole of depression and some are left contemplating for themselves the very act that took their own child.

GROUPS AT AN ELEVATED RISK FOR SUICIDE

Suicide patterns among groups have been carefully studied. A report from the surgeon general reveals that suicide is highly correlated with mental illness and substance abuse. Suicide is also more common among American Indians and Alaska natives. In addition, gay, lesbian, bisexual, and transgender populations are at higher risk for suicide, as are individuals coping with a loved one's death. Their risk increases if that person's death was due to suicide. Individuals who engage in self-harmful behaviors such as cutting are more likely than the rest of the population to eventually commit suicide.

Numerous media reports have covered the high rates of suicide among active duty Armed Forces and military veterans. The rates have remained high despite intensive efforts by military medicine and the Veterans Administration (VA) to help these young soldiers. A recent report from the VA indicates that although the percentage of veterans who died from suicide has slightly fallen since 1999, the actual numbers of deaths from suicide has risen since then. The VA has initiated a Veterans Crisis Line (800-273-8255, push 1) for suicidal veterans, or individuals can text 838255 to contact the VA.

Suicide is also a prevalent problem for those incarcerated in jails and prisons and for patients with serious medical conditions, particularly cancer. According to the National Institute of Mental Health (NIMH), having highly conflicted and violent relationships with others also elevates the risk for suicide. Other risk factors include a personal history of physical or sexual abuse and the presence of firearms in the home.

MENTAL ILLNESS, SUBSTANCE ABUSE, AND SUICIDE

When psychiatrists ponder a patient's suicidal behavior, they also immediately evaluate whether mental illness is present. High rates of suicide attempts have been identified among those with bipolar disorder, followed by individuals with major depression. In addition, alcoholism, drug addiction, and other mental health diagnoses increase the risk for suicide.

Psychiatric Illness, Alcoholism, and the Risk for Suicide

In a 2011 publication, Leonard Tondo, MD, and Ross J. Baldessarini, MD, analyzed the results of 28 studies involving 21,500 patients with bipolar disorder. Of these patients, 823 died from suicide, a rate of 390 per 100,000 individuals. This rate is 26 times greater than the risk for suicide in a general population, a prevalence that was surprisingly high.

Other psychiatric illnesses are linked to suicide. The results of a landmark Mexican study of nearly 6,000 subjects drawn from the Mexican National Comorbidity Survey was published in the *Journal of Affective Disorders* in 2010. The researchers found that nearly half of the subjects with suicidal thoughts had previously been diagnosed with a psychiatric disorder. Of those who had attempted suicide, nearly two-thirds had a known psychiatric disorder. The strongest predictors for another suicide attempt were a diagnosis of conduct disorder (a disorder of defying authority and acting out) or alcohol abuse or dependence. The presence of either condition increased the risk for a suicide attempt by six times. The next most serious predictor for suicide was the presence of an anxiety disorder, which increased the risk of another suicide attempt by two to three times greater than among those without anxiety disorders.

WHY YOU SHOULD INTERVENE AND WHAT YOU CAN DO

When they learn of their child's despair, most parents would do anything to reverse the situation for their adult child. Others are paralyzed by the gravity of the situation or meet their child's crisis with a sense of resignation. Most families are relieved to learn that doctors and families can decrease the risk of losing an adult child to suicide.

Psychiatric Treatment

Psychiatric treatment is proven to reduce the frequency and intensity of suicidal thinking. This finding is best exemplified by studies concerning lithium carbonate, the standard psychiatric treatment for bipolar disorder. In various studies, treatment with lithium significantly lowered the risk of suicide. Patients taking lithium had nearly a three times lower rate of suicide than patients who were taking other bipolar medications. Another study uncovered that the risk for suicide increased by twenty-fold *after* the discontinuation of lithium and a rapid discontinuation of the medication rather than a slow tapering of the dose. The studies cemented the belief that lithium has antisuicidal properties.

Schizophrenia, as with bipolar disorder, carries a high risk of suicide. People with schizophrenia have an 8.5 times greater risk of suicide compared to the risk among the general population. Yet treatment with the antipsychotic clozapine has demonstrated significantly reduced rates of suicide to the extent that the FDA approved the medication for this specific indication.

Treatment for drug and alcohol dependency also lowers the risk for suicide. Rates of suicide decline during periods of sobriety from alcohol or drugs. Not all who suffer from these conditions will welcome treatment, but if they are treated, they lessen the chance of death at their own hands.

Family Intervention

If your adult child describes suicidal thoughts to you, it is essential to reach out to her and to encourage her that hope still exists. For example, help your child make contact with a doctor. Offer to drive them to their appointments. Usually suicidal thoughts pass quickly, and cushioning your loved one who is in the depths of the crisis can help to avert disaster.

Suicide is often an impulsive act, and if you can get your child past the immediate danger zone, you might outrun the threat. Paul S. F. Yipp and colleagues report that suicide attempts are often spur of the moment decisions. If a lethal means of committing suicide is unavailable, then the suicide attempt may be delayed, and hopefully the suicidal impulse will not recur. This reasoning holds for individuals in crisis and those who have recurrent suicidal thoughts.

The best way to protect homes with suicidal family members is to remove guns and other weapons. By placing obstacles in their adult child's way, families may have given him a second chance, and it also gives the family one more opportunity to get him treatment. The goal is to postpone and avert a crisis. You can never assume that the problem is totally

---

SHE LIVES WITH HER SUICIDAL DAUGHTER

Audrey has always been a troubled girl. In grade school, she was diagnosed with ADHD. Then in middle school, she developed an eating disorder. In her late teenage years, she was diagnosed with bipolar disorder. She is now age twenty-four and her most recent therapist diagnosed her with borderline personality disorder.

The only thing stable about Audrey is that she is consistently unstable. At every turn, Audrey has had problems. She was unable to complete her public school education. Every intimate relationship she has is rocky and always ends poorly. Audrey also overreacts to mundane frustrations, lambasting her family and quickly becoming suicidal when she becomes frustrated. Sometimes Audrey acts on these self-destructive impulses. Recently after her work hours were reduced, she superficially cut her wrists with an Exacto knife.

The hospital emergency center bandaged Audrey's wounds and no sutures were required. A few months later, she left home in a rage after an argument with her parents. A policeman happened to notice Audrey unconscious in her car, and rushed her to the hospital. Mercifully, Audrey's overdose was not lethal, but when she woke up the next day, she could not understand everyone's distress, and said, "I had no intention to kill myself."

Parents can develop intense and very uncomfortable feelings about their chronically suicidal children. In an interview at the hospital, Audrey's mother conceded, "When Audrey is suicidal, sometimes I wish that she would just do it, so the temper tantrums, emotional abuse, and my worrying would be over. She says that sometimes she wishes I would die too. But neither one of us wants to live without the other in the world. We sometimes laugh about our conflicted feelings."

---

over, of course, nor should you believe that suicide and death are inevitable for your child. Instead take an adversarial stance against the forces bringing your child down.

Maintain a Proactive Attitude

For those with chronic depression, suicidal thoughts are ongoing and exhausting. When the thoughts become more intense, hopelessness may set in, and your child may assert that medications or therapy are both futile actions. The truth is that anyone who contemplates suicide once, particularly if their treatment is disrupted, is likely to find herself in that bad, dark place again. It is important for you not to adopt the same sense of hopelessness.

You might agree with your child that some past treatments have been disappointing. In the tension of the moment, however, it is best not to engage in this discussion. At those moments, families need to physically separate their child from guns, pills, and other dangers. This might require voluntary hospitalization and it is always best to do this with your child's consent. However, without their consent, an involuntary hospitalization, committing your child to a psychiatric facility against his will because he is a danger to himself, may need to be a consideration. This difficult process of involuntary hospitalization will be discussed later in the chapter.

Take Suicide Threats Seriously

Always take suicide threats seriously. If your adult child says she has a plan or is going to kill herself now, it may be a real threat or just another means to manipulate you to do something. However, never assume that the threat is not real. This could be a fatal mistake.

PREDICTORS FOR RECURRENT SUICIDAL BEHAVIOR

If a person like Audrey (see She Lives with Her Suicidal Daughter) tries to commit suicide once, will she try it again? This section covers the risk factors that have been shown to predict the likelihood of suicide attempts. Factors that guard against suicidal behavior are also explored.

A 2012 report from the surgeon general has identified a number of known behaviors that are associated with a future risk for suicide. The greater the number of these signs that are present in a person, then the higher the risk is for suicide in that individual.

- The person has a specific plan for suicide.
- The person has attempted suicide in the past.

- The person has access to the means to commit suicide, such as pills that could cause death or a gun.

- The person is suddenly cheerful after a long depression.

- The individual was recently placed on antidepressants.

- The individual has intensified his use of alcohol or drugs, or of both alcohol and drugs.

- The individual has reported an increase in the intensity of command hallucinations (in individuals previously diagnosed with a psychotic illness). The internal voices may urge the person to commit suicide.

The Person Has a Specific Suicide Plan

The presence of a specific suicide plan signals danger. Talking about wanting to die or developing a plan detailing when or how the act will occur increases the concern that a person may act on her suicidal ideas.

The Person Has Attempted Suicide in the Past

Unfortunately, the past is often prologue to the future. When a person has attempted suicide in the past, he is at an increased risk for a future attempt. Several factors contribute to this finding, but the most likely is that suicidal behavior occurs during periods of depression. Under the best circumstances, it is hard to live with a mood disorder. If your child loses his job or relationship during an episode of depression, the risk of suicide increases.

The Person Has the Means to Commit Suicide

Most suicides involve guns or an overdose of pills. Restrict these means, whenever possible. Suicide is often an impulsive act, and at-risk individuals should not have easy access to the means that are used for suicide. Some families of troubled children avoid housing any firearms, and if they own guns, they are kept offsite. Families who are uncomfortable with this option should ensure that any guns they own at home are kept in a secure locked cabinet that cannot be broken into by their adult child. The key or the safe combination should remain with the owner only, not in an obvious place, and the bullets should be stored separately.

Similarly, many medications are dangerous in overdose and large reserves should not be kept in the homes of loved ones with recurrent depression. Opiate medications are lethal in overdose, and unused prescription painkillers should be locked up or safely discarded. Even over the counter medications like Tylenol should be available only in small amounts.

There are many other methods to perform suicide. Parents lose their children to hanging, drowning, jumping off high sites, and carbon monoxide poisoning. You cannot protect against all these factors, and you can only be vigilant that the threat exists.

The Individual Is Suddenly Cheerful

Doctors have noted that rapid mood swings are common in suicidal patients. There are also reports of severely depressed patients becoming suddenly cheerful, a switch that makes their subsequent suicidal attempt seem even more shocking. Some experts speculate that this shift signifies that the person has now resolved to commit suicide, and that he feels comfortable with the decision.

The Person Was Recently Placed on Antidepressants

A small percentage of depressed individuals taking antidepressant medications may have a brief period of increased suicidal risk soon after starting their medication. It is believed that these medications may give the depressed person the energy to act on their negative feelings. The risk is greater among individuals younger than twenty-five years old. The FDA has mandated that this warning be included in all packaging for antidepressants. Although this paradoxical reaction is uncommon, the black box has had the unfortunate consequence of discouraging many doctors from using antidepressants in younger patients.

The Psychotic Person Hears Voices Telling Her to Commit Suicide

Suicide is associated with both depression and psychosis. Auditory hallucinations (hearing voices) are the hallmark symptom of schizophrenia, a psychotic disorder. An increase in command hallucinations, which refers to internal voices that issue orders to the person, may herald the onset of suicidal behavior. Many patients suffer for years from these terrifying hallucinations, but the overwhelming majority never act on the harsh directions. Command hallucinations are most likely to return after stopping antipsychotic medications.

Protective Factors against Suicide

There are some factors that protect against suicide. Patients do better if they have access to physical and mental health care. Follow-up care after a psychiatric hospitalization is essential, as is a sense of connectedness to family, friends, and the community. Everyone needs self-defined reasons for living. Beyond all this, perhaps nothing protects your adult child from suicide more than the knowledge that their own children need them.

WARNING SIGNS OF SUICIDE

- Talking about wanting to die
- Looking for a way to kill oneself
- Talking about feeling hopeless or having no purpose
- Talking about feeling trapped or being in unbearable pain
- Talking about being a burden to others
- Increasing the use of alcohol or drugs
- Acting anxious, agitated, or restless
- Sleeping too little or too much
- Withdrawing or feeling isolated
- Showing rage or talking about seeking revenge
- Displaying extreme mood swings

WHAT TO DO IF YOU SUSPECT THAT YOUR ADULT CHILD IS SUICIDAL

Parents can take the following actions if they see troubling signs of a possible suicidal intent within their adult child:

- Do not leave your child alone.
- Develop a relationship with your child's doctor.
- Call the police.
- Consider hospitalization for your adult child.

Do Not Leave Your Suicidal Child Alone

Usually suicidal impulses come and go. When your adult child is in the depths of a crisis, stay with him. If you cannot be there, then arrange for another family member or a friend to be present with your child. Of course, no family can stand vigil forever. When a longer-term solution is required, then a hospital stay may be in order. If you think that your child is a risk to himself and/or to others, then contact the police and tell them so. Provide clear examples of what you are concerned about. Be sure to state that your adult child is a danger to himself and needs to be protected from his own suicidal impulses.

Develop a Relationship with Your Child's Therapist

If your adult child is chronically suicidal, try to develop a working relationship with your child's therapist. If you have built rapport during periods of relative calm, then you have a partner who can help you in a time of crisis. It is wise to have a release of information agreement signed by your adult child ensuring that you legally can talk to her doctor and that the doctor can answer back freely. Without this release, the doctor cannot provide you with confidential information, although she can act on information that you offer. During periods of crisis the doctor will be able to guide you about appropriate actions to take.

Call the Police

The role of the police in urgent situations is not to treat your loved one's psychiatric condition, but rather to protect him and to help solve the imminent problem. If you think your adult child is in imminent danger of suicide, contact the police and inform them of the emergency situation. The police have both the might and the mobility to come to your home in

---

**CALL THE US NATIONAL SUICIDE PREVENTION LIFELINE
AT (800) 273-8255**

The National Suicide Prevention Lifeline is an important number to store in
your phone. You might be having a hard time deciding what to do in such a
major crisis, and these experts can help guide you through this very difficult
time.

---

a crisis. Police are aware of local commitment laws and will be willing and
able to take the individual to the emergency room for assessment.

Be very forthcoming with information if the police come to your
home. If your child is in a psychotic state and is threatening you, let them
know. If you find a suicide note, then provide the police with a copy. Never
give up the original note—it may be useful later in the commitment process or as a piece of evidence.

Consider Hospitalization

You may need to consider hospitalization to avert the risk for suicide.
The hospital staff can evaluate the situation and provide physical safety
temporarily in the emergency department until the short crisis passes, or
by admitting your child to a psychiatric unit. Some suicidal behaviors are
more ominous than others, but in the crush of the moment, it is very helpful to get the input of an experienced staff with appropriate resources at
their disposal.

Once your child is in the hospital, you should seek to partner with the
doctors as much as possible. Ask your child's psychiatrist to contact the
hospital doctors to provide them with information. Working together, a
good decision about any further steps that need to be taken can be made.

As mentioned elsewhere in the book, doctors may refuse to provide
you with information. But they are not prohibited from listening to what
you have to say and choosing to act (or not) on it. They will likely not
tell you what they have decided because of privacy regulations. But your
insights may be very valuable to the doctors.

Most of the time, an individual with suicidal thoughts will voluntarily sign herself into a psychiatric hospital. However, sometimes your child might push back and refuse inpatient treatment. At these times, the option of an involuntarily hospitalization becomes an important consideration.

Involuntary Hospitalization for Suicidal or Aggressive Behavior

Each state has its own particular legal criteria for the circumstances under which an involuntary admission to a psychiatric unit may be made. The general rule for an involuntary commitment is that the individual must be a credible and imminent threat to himself or to others. The process of civil commitment varies by state, but it generally follows a logical pattern. In Michigan, for example, a *petition* is a legal statement that is completed by people who have witnessed the individual's suicidal or aggressive behavior.

Petitions to the court detail the concerning behavior and are usually completed by a therapist, family, or friend. A psychiatrist, physician, or licensed psychologist may also sign a *civil certification* essentially confirming the threat. With these two elements, the patient is confined to the hospital involuntarily for at least seventy-two hours. During this time, the patient may sign in on a voluntary basis or be offered an attorney to challenge the commitment.

When a person is civilly committed, the hospital determines the level of the person's dangerousness. If experts at the facility do not believe that the person is a threat to himself or others anymore, then he will be discharged. However, if they acknowledge that the person needs hospitalization, and if a longer treatment is deemed necessary, the court has the power to order further treatment until the immediate danger recedes. The patient may be discharged with the stipulation that he receive outpatient psychiatric care.

SURVIVING YOUR ADULT CHILD'S SUICIDE

Probably the most difficult experience imaginable is to survive your own child's suicide. This act causes an emotional pain that lasts indefinitely, although the most intense pain occurs shortly after the suicide and for about a year afterwards. Parents wonder what they could have done to prevent the suicide and have many "if-onlys." If only they had called the child on that day or had done something else differently, they think, maybe they could have prevented it. If only they had told him that he was loved, maybe he would have stopped before going through with the suicide. If the last words with the child were words of anger, this is yet another cause for regret.

Stages of Bereavement

Many years ago, Elisabeth Kübler-Ross, a brilliant psychiatrist, described five general stages of grieving that may occur when a person suffers a severe loss. A diagnosis of terminal cancer or the death of a family member may trigger psychological reactions known as denial, anger, bargaining, depression, and acceptance. These stages do not always occur in sequence, and some people experience some stages and not others.

Denial

When a child dies at his own hand, the shock of the experience may be too overwhelming to grasp. It is normal for a mother or father to deny that it possibly *could* have happened. Denial is not a wrong or bad reaction and it gives a person a chance to process this terrible news.

Anger

Many parents become angry when they learn of their child's suicide. They may be angry with the child's doctor for not having prevented the suicide. They may be angry with others who they felt did not take the situation as seriously as it clearly was. They may be irrationally angry at many different people. If they are religious individuals, they may be angry with God for allowing the suicide to occur and not having stopped it at the last moment. They may also be angry with their child for ending his life. When a mother gives birth to her child, she has many hopes and dreams for him. When he ends his life, it may seem like a repudiation of that person's life.

Bargaining

If the child has not died from suicide but is in clear danger of death because of her suicidal tendencies, the parent may try to bargain with God or the doctor. For example, the parent praying to God to please save her child and she will forever after go to church faithfully unless she can't because she's in the hospital, or begging the doctor to save her child and she'll do volunteer work for his favorite charity. Of the many other types of bargaining, some are verbalized and some are not.

Depression

When you lose someone you love, especially your own child, depression may be inevitable. Throughout the country, support groups such as Compassionate Friends welcome survivors of suicide. Most are survivors themselves. If depression lingers and is debilitating, consultation with a psychiatrist may be needed. Therapy and antidepressants can help considerably with symptoms of grief.

Acceptance

It is hard to fully accept the fate of an adult child who commits suicide. Feelings of emptiness will inevitably be mixed with feelings of anger. Loss may alternate with relief, especially if your child was long troubled. Grief waxes and wanes and abates only with time. It comes back again at certain times, rawness covered by the passage of time.

Parents React Strongly to Their Adult Child's Suicide

Dr. Kübler-Ross's famous stages led to empirical research on survivors of suicide. In a large study, James M. Bolton, MD, and colleagues compared adults whose children had died from suicide (1,415 subjects) to parents bereaved by their child's death from a car crash (1,132 subjects) and to nonbereaved parents (also 1,415 subjects).

The researchers found that suicide bereavement in parents was associated with an elevated rate of depression, anxiety disorders, and marital failure within two years after the suicide had occurred. They also found that suicide bereavement was also associated with an increased risk for mental illness hospitalization among the parents when they were compared to the other groups. The subjects in the suicide bereavement group were also more likely to suffer from physical disorders, such as cancer, hypertension, and diabetes than the subjects in the other groups.

In addition, the parents bereaved by suicide had an increased risk for alcohol use disorders both before and after the death of their child, a risk more than three times greater than found among the nonbereaved group of parents.

Clearly, the loss of a child through suicide has a profound effect on parents, and this subject should be studied further, not only to understand further how suicide affects parents but also to ascertain how mental health professionals, physicians, and the friends and family of bereaved individuals can better help them.

OUTCOMES OF CASES IN THIS CHAPTER

So what happened in the cases of Cole, Audrey, and Michael, all suicidal, and described in this chapter? Cole had a good outcome. He allowed his mother to get him professional help and he started to see a psychiatric nurse practitioner for therapy. Cole also responded well to an antidepressant medication. Through therapy, Cole began to accept his sexuality, and he recognized that the extreme lengths that he had gone to in order to pretend to be straight, particularly marrying a straight woman, had caused him great internal conflict and depression. Cole and Michelle divorced amicably and his suicidal thoughts did not recur.

Audrey improved over time. A new psychiatrist viewed Audrey's behavior as impulsive and diagnosed her with ADHD. Treatment with a long-acting stimulant medication muted Audrey's rapid mood swings. Audrey returned to school, and she also found a part-time job she enjoyed. Her suicidal thoughts and actions became rarer and eventually abated.

Tragically, Marie never made contact with her son Michael in time. After she read his e-mail, Marie frantically called the police and her son's landlord. The landlord found him first; Michael had hung himself the night before. Years later, Marie's wounds heal ever so slowly.

KEY POINTS IN THIS CHAPTER

- Suicidal behaviors may include suicidal ideas, gestures, failed attempts, and "completed" suicide attempts that result in death.

- Parents whose children attempt or complete a suicide suffer severe stages of grief.

- If you think that your child is suicidal, then you need to act. For example, be with your child or have someone else be with her, and get rid of any means to kill herself, such as guns or knives.

- There are predictors for a suicide attempt, such as a prior attempt, substance abuse, or psychiatric problems.

It is easy to forget in the midst of crisis, and especially when one crisis seems to closely follow another, but it is also very important to take care of yourself when you have an adult child who has severe issues. That is the subject of Part Three.

Part Three

Taking Care of Yourself

This part covers the importance of tending to your own psychological and physical health when you are also concerned about severe issues with your adult child.

CHAPTER 9
YOUR PHYSICAL AND EMOTIONAL HEALTH

Lorraine felt her heart pounding and her anxiety level rising. Her son T. J., age twenty-five, was in trouble again and he needed money right away. He said if Lorraine did not pay his rent, then he would be in violation of his probation and would be at the mercy of the courts. Lorraine didn't want T. J. to go to prison—she knew terrible things could happen to him there. But she didn't have much money left, and she was concerned about paying her own bills. Now her head was aching and her stomach started hurting too. She couldn't stand this situation much longer.

The stress of having a troubled adult child can affect your physical and emotional health, and it also magnifies the flaws in a marital relationship. Lorraine and her husband had drastically different approaches to T. J. Lorraine believed that parents should do anything to help their children and that her selfless love was a basic instinct. Her connection to T. J. started with his first breath and she never lost the feeling even as he grew older and less innocent.

Her husband Bill deeply resented the constant pressure that T. J. placed on the family. Bill frequently reminded Lorraine that their son was now an adult, and he needed to make his own way in life without extracting pounds of emotional and financial flesh from his parents. From his earlier school expulsions and vandalism to his later alcohol binges, they had seen it all and it seemed like they never stopped fighting with each other about what they should do. Bill's anger indiscriminately extended to both his son and wife. The agony of watching T. J. self-destruct, coupled with her husband's furious anger, compounded Lorraine's despair and worsened her physical symptoms of stomach pain and headaches. She was torn between the two men in her life and she wanted to be strong for both of them. To do so, she knew that she had to make good decisions about herself.

ATTEND TO YOUR OWN PHYSICAL HEALTH NEEDS

Each phase of life is attached to unique challenges, and in general, your capabilities usually match what is demanded of you. For example, small children are physically active but they are usually not concerned about the consequences of careless behavior. They frequently fall down and suffer scraped knees, but their bodies are light and they can recover and heal.

Adults in their thirties and forties (and older) face the dual challenge of guiding their teenagers through adolescence and their parents through old age. They adapt because generally they have sufficient energy and wisdom of age to address the needs of both ends of the life spectrum. This convenient coupling of demand and capability reaches its limit when older parents are forced to deal with their troubled adult children. The parents who best survive the emotional pressures are those who address their own physical and emotional health. This section covers your physical health.

Take Care of Yourself

However consuming your adult children may be in your life, be sure to pay attention to your own health care needs. A good place to start is by creating a relationship with a primary care provider, if you don't have one. Or, if you do have a doctor, but you haven't seen her for a year or more because of the demands of your children, make an appointment. Under the care of a family doctor or a nurse practitioner, you can structure a program to maintain your weight, control your blood pressure, and manage your cholesterol and lipids. Implementing a rational exercise program and smart diet will also help to promote your well-being.

There is even more reason to ally with a doctor if you have underlying health problems. Conditions such as hypertension, diabetes, and obesity will intensify if not properly managed. Under constant stress, it is easy to drop your guard and forget to watch your caloric intake or to take your medications. Pay particular attention to your sleep cycle. People tend to worry more at night when pleasant distractions subside and the house quiets down. Inform your doctor if you experience insomnia or daytime fatigue. These conditions, as well as snoring that is associated

---

PHYSICAL SYMPTOMS ARE COMMON WITH TOUGH TIMES

Andrea relates the following story to her therapist. "When things get really bad with our daughter, she always turns to us. She calls me at least once a day and depends on us to bail her out of every problem. We end up paying her car insurance and her credit card bills. My husband seethes every time her bad decisions cost money. He gets bad headaches and I just eat and eat. I have gained twenty-five pounds in the last few years. When she's in crisis, we fall apart."

---

with obstructive sleep apnea, are treatable, and improvement in these symptoms will help you to fortify your health during difficult times.

Take Care of Existing Health Problems

If you already have health problems, these problems may worsen when you are distressed by your adult child's problems. For example, if you have hypertension and/or type 2 diabetes, you may forget to take your medication, risking a dangerous rise in your blood pressure or your blood glucose. You may lose sleep, night after night, as you try to figure out how to solve your adult child's problems. But often there is no obvious Aha! solution to such difficult problems as mental illness, substance abuse, and criminal behavior. Maybe you want your adult child to get treated by a psychiatrist, but she refuses, insisting that there is nothing wrong with her, further raising your blood pressure.

Take a look at the chart on page 165 to see how some chronic health problems can become worse when you are struggling to help your adult child with her issues and ignoring your own health.

CONSIDER YOUR EMOTIONAL HEALTH

People who control their blood pressure are less likely to die of a stroke and those who keep their cholesterol under 200 reduce their risk of heart disease. These are very meaningful goals, but the payoff is years down the road rather than now. In contrast, if you experience anxiety or depression,

Why Some Health Problems Get Worse When You're Upset

Health Problem	What May Happen/Not Happen If You Get Upset	Possible Consequences of Your Actions/Inactions
You have diabetes.	You may not take your medications. You may fail to test your blood sugar.	Your blood sugar goes up. You risk problems with the heart, kidneys, eyes (blindness), and other organs.
You have hypertension.	You may fail to take your antihypertensive medicine or check your blood pressure.	Your blood pressure escalates. You risk a stroke or a heart attack.
Your thyroid levels are low or otherwise abnormal.	You may skip your blood test for your thyroid levels and miss your appointment with your doctor.	You risk over- or underactive thyroid activity, which may make you feel lethargic (if you are hypothyroid) or extremely nervous (if you are hyperthyroid). You need to get the blood test and see the doctor to interpret the test results for you.
You have had cancer in the past several years.	You cancel your appointment with your oncologist because everyone dies and you're too busy helping your adult child.	If cancer recurs, often it can be treated. But it has to be identified by your doctor in a timely manner to be treated.
You are obese.	You may decide that you need a few more cookies every day to cope with your distress over your adult child.	You gain weight and increase your risk for type 2 diabetes, hypertension, cancer, and other illnesses.
You have a few drinks of alcohol every night.	You decide an extra few drinks couldn't hurt.	You are wrong. Heavy drinking can lead to many diseases and disorders. Not only do you risk developing alcoholism, but you also risk getting liver disease, cancer, and other major health problems.

you are suffering in real time. You want relief immediately. Symptoms of depression and anxiety can emerge out of the blue, but usually they result from stressful circumstances. These conditions also run in families and some people are genetically predisposed to getting depressed.

Depression and anxiety haunt the lives of parents of adult children with serious issues. Parents may become depressed because their adult child keeps getting into trouble. They may become anxious because they anticipate another sorrowful predicament will arise without warning. They can't escape their questions and the self-doubt. What if she gets into an accident or hurts someone? What if he goes back to jail? Where will she go if she's evicted? Where did we go wrong?

Parents of troubled adult children ask these questions in search of honest answers. But just as you want your adult children to get treatment to allow them to function at their best, so might you also need to seek professional help if you become severely anxious or depressed.

Current treatments for anxiety and depression involve medications and psychotherapy. Newer medications can reverse symptoms, often quite quickly. But unless the symptoms are quite severe, many parents elect to "talk it out" in therapy. Often a blend of therapy and medications is the preferred route to help parents of adult children with issues. Therapy is to medication what salt (in moderation!) is to french fries. They are much better together than alone.

Be Honest with the Psychiatrist or Other Therapist

If you do see a mental health professional, in your first session you will provide some background information about yourself and possibly of your childhood. You may have brought in a sheet about your medical issues and any medications you take that you filled out before your session.

The psychiatrist (or therapist) will try to put you at ease. He knows that many people are nervous at first. Then you will describe your problem to him as you see it. You may think, for example, that you are depressed and so you tell the psychiatrist/therapist why you are depressed. He may agree with you about the depression, or he may think that your problem could be another issue altogether. For example, if you are very agitated, the psychiatrist/therapist may consider that you have an anxiety disorder. Or maybe you have both an anxiety disorder and depression; often those two issues go together. You could also have adult attention-deficit disorder (ADHD). There are many other possibilities. Listen to the psychiatrist/therapist when he explains his diagnosis and the treatment he recommends.

Listen to Her Suggestions and Try to Follow Them

The psychiatrist may recommend that you try a medication, such as an anti-anxiety medication or an antidepressant, or if you are seeing a therapist he may refer you to a psychiatrist. If medications are recommended, often the doctor starts you on a low dosage of the drug, which may be increased later. The doctor will also take into account any other medications that you take now because she does not want to risk a possible drug interaction, or the side effects that can occur when you take two drugs that do not go well together. Medication interactions may be minor, but sometimes they are serious. For example, one form of antidepressant, the MAO inhibitor, must not be taken with some other drugs because of possible serious interactions. Many psychiatrists don't prescribe this drug anymore because it has so many interactions, but your doctor may feel like the MAO inhibitor could really help you.

The psychiatrist will also likely offer you suggestions. For example, he may recommend that you receive therapy with another person who is a psychologist. He may also offer you advice on dealing with your adult child. If it makes sense to you, then try to follow it.

Tell Your Primary Care Doctor about Any Medication Changes

You don't have to share your diagnosis or anything else that you told your psychiatrist or that he told you. But if medication is prescribed for you, then you do need to tell your family practitioner or internist. The reason for this is the same reason why you needed to tell the psychiatrist about medications that you currently take. Your primary care doctor needs to know about medications that other doctors order so that he doesn't risk prescribing a medication in the future that could have an interaction with the new drug.

TYPES OF THERAPY

There are several different types of therapy mental health professionals may use to help the parents of adult children with issues. Keep in mind that many of the rules of psychotherapy have changed over time. Gone is the era of psychoanalysis when a patient lay on a couch three times a week while his analyst dissected minute behavior and explored the person's early childhood. Much time was spent recollecting the patient's parents' behavior and this frequently led to faulty conclusions, such as, "Your mother was too involved with her vanity over her beauty, hence you are now an anxious and insecure adult."

Although all therapists concede that the experiences of childhood play an important role in the person we become, many current psychological treatments focus on the present, not the past. Two of the most common treatment strategies, supportive therapy and cognitive behavioral therapy (CBT), are described in this section. Understanding these different approaches allows you to seek help from a therapist whose healing philosophy aligns with yours.

Supportive Therapy

Supportive therapies are the most widely available; they borrow heavily from traditional psychodynamic principles but also readily integrate other schools of thought into practice. This eclectic approach emphasizes that emotional relief comes from establishing a safe and warm relationship between the therapist and patient. Good supportive therapists are active listeners and good questioners who do not shy away from making pragmatic interpretations.

Remember Andrea, described earlier in a sidebar in this chapter? She was hesitant at first about therapy, and only after coaxing from a friend did she decide to seek help. Andrea found the website of an established local mental health clinic that accepted her health insurance. Each of the therapists had a brief biography and a short description of their treatment philosophy. Andrea chose to see a social worker with whom she shared a similar background.

Andrea was instantly comfortable with Marie. Both were Italian, in their early fifties, and came from immigrant families. This initial comfort allowed for an instant alliance and a productive conversation. Marie felt that the first order of business was addressing her overwhelming anxiety, and she arranged for Andrea to see the clinic psychiatrist the next day. The doctor diagnosed Andrea with panic disorder and prescribed medications that helped her within a few days. Relieved of the incapacitating panic and grateful for Marie's intervention, Andrea was encouraged to barrel ahead in her therapy.

At their next sessions, Andrea opened up about her marriage to Doug, a successful pharmacist and businessman. She lamented their loss of intimacy over the last few years. Andrea said, "We stop talking to each other for days at a time—usually when my daughter makes bad judgments or spends too much money. He is a man of few words, but when he gets angry now, he starts to sweat and become flushed. "

Marie commented, "This seems to deeply affect you."

Andrea continued, "Yes when this happens, I just back off and do something to stay busy. This means that I do a lot of baking and eating. I think I just eat to avoid worrying."

Marie pushed the issue. "You shared with me that that your husband was a wealthy man and your daughter's overspending is not a real burden to him. Maybe there is something more going on here than the problems your daughter creates."

Andrea was intrigued, and Marie continued, "You seem to view your husband as a very disabled person—someone who is ready to drop over anytime. You have become so fearful, that any time your daughter appears, you think he is going to have a stroke. You are reacting to her foolish decisions and, more severely, to the way you think it affects your husband's health. But is he really that fragile?"

Andrea returned to therapy two weeks later and was eager to share new information with Marie. "Because we talked about this at our last session, I was able to tell Doug that I was worried about his health. He allowed me to go with him to his cardiologist. The doctor said he checked out fine and had a healthy heart. He was sweating and flushing because of a medication side effect. The doctor changed his medication and he is fine."

The good news allowed Andrea to feel more confident about Doug's well-being. "For the first time in a long time, I don't feel like he is going to die tomorrow. I had become like a nurse or aide rather than his wife."

A few sessions later Marie asked the next natural question. "How has this new knowledge affected your sex life?"

Andrea responded, "I admit it took me a while, but we are back on track. We have sex now and Doug is much happier. He was frustrated and sad that I had stopped treating him as a desirable person. Nothing is perfect, but as we get along better as a couple, we are again starting to meet each other's needs. When we worked through our own issues, our former constant harping about our daughter's problems lessened."

In this case, both therapist and patient felt that supportive therapy helped the family.

Cognitive Behavioral Therapy (CBT)

Cognitive behavioral therapy is one of the most proven psychological treatments. It has been studied in the treatment of various conditions ranging from insomnia to eating disorders, although CBT is most commonly employed for the treatment of anxiety and depression. A typical CBT treatment consists of six to eighteen meetings with a trained therapist, typically with one week between sessions. The patient is sent home with cognitive exercises to perform between sessions to further reinforce the principles learned within sessions. The therapist may also encourage the individual to try new or avoided behaviors to bring about change. The therapy was developed by Aaron T. Beck and Albert Ellis. Dr. David Burns and other therapists and writers have modified CBT principles to make them easily applicable to patients.

CBT focuses on the underlying thoughts behind an individual's feelings. CBT holds that reviewing one's past is not necessary for healing. Instead, patients need to identify their current personal patterns of distorted thinking. By correcting these cognitive distortions, patients will no longer misperceive their environment and they will feel better.

The cognitive therapist listens carefully to you to discern your patterns of thinking. She will note your concerns and evaluate whether you are processing the information logically. If you have distorted thinking, she will identify the type of distorted thinking that is applicable in your case, and will teach you how to replace these distortions with more rational thoughts. Armed with appropriate replacement thoughts, individuals will have less anxiety and depression. CBT retrains your thoughts so that you do not fall into old, counterproductive patterns. The goal of CBT is to allow you to ultimately trust your own reasoning.

CBT CASE STUDY: SYLVIA AND HER DAUGHTER

Sylvia, sixty-four, was referred to Dr. M, an experienced CBT therapist, for help with her relationship with her adult daughter. Dr. M started the treatment by encouraging Sylvia to provide some background about her current problems. Dr. M said, "I want to understand the context before we start working on issues."

Sylvia agreed and told her story. She had raised Jane (now age forty) and her brother Sam after their father died in a car accident when Jane was three and Sam was five. Finances were tight, and Sylvia worked several jobs to keep her family afloat. She recalls feeling continually exhausted throughout her children's upbringing, and, in retrospect she also admits to being very depressed after her husband's death.

Sylvia remarried when her children were in their teens. Her husband was distant from the children and generally resented their demands on Sylvia's time. Sylvia did her best to make sure her children participated in activities like sports, music, and after school clubs. She also attended parent conferences and school fundraisers. After her divorce, the pressure of supporting the family often conflicted with Sylvia's parenting time. She was not available as much as she would have liked to help them with homework and enjoy the fun times.

When Jane was a teenager, she became moody and aloof. Jane dated boys who did not respect her and she became increasingly insecure with each new relationship. Jane admitted to having sex with one boy who threatened to break up with her if she did not acquiesce to his demand for sex. When Sylvia tried to limit her exposure to this boy, Jane threatened to move out of the house if Sylvia interfered. Sylvia sought counseling for herself and Jane, but Jane refused to go. Sylvia desperately wanted her daughter to finish high school and start college where she could get a fresh start and increase her chances of a bright future. Sylvia did her best to keep peace in the house and she shied away from conflict.

Jane completed high school as Sylvia wished, but her performance was lackluster at best. She lacked ambition to go to college and continued a long string of failed relationships with men. Jane worked at minimum wage jobs, but was often fired for failing to show up on time or calling in sick. She constantly complained about having insufficient finances and looked to Sylvia to help her move to a different apartment, pay back loans, and buy her new clothes for job interviews.

Identifying Automatic Thoughts

Dr. M asked Sylvia, "It sounds like this has been a struggle for a long time. Why did you decide to get help now?

SYLVIA: "Because I am at the breaking point. Jane called a few weeks ago, asking for a $2,000 loan to fix her boyfriend's truck. This guy has gone to jail for writing forged checks and owes thousands of dollars in child support to his first wife. Without the loan, Jane thinks his new lawn business will fail. She hopes once his business takes off, they could buy a house, get married, and start a family."

DR. M: "What do you think would happen if you did not give her the money?"

SYLVIA: "I don't know. I did not really trust him and I doubt that I would ever see the money again. But I did get a loan from my credit union and gave them the money anyway."

Dr. M tried to help Sylvia identify her automatic thoughts when she first received Jane's request.

SYLVIA: "My instinct was to get the money to her. I told myself that it really wasn't that much money and if this would give her stability, then I was willing to make the sacrifice."

Dr. M interpreted Sylvia's thinking pattern. It appeared that Sylvia's thoughts generated feelings of guilt for bringing up Jane without a stable father. She also regretted that she couldn't provide amenities for her daughter growing up. She made comments to herself such as, "If I had been a better parent, wouldn't Jane now be living a stable, middle class life with a husband and two children in the suburbs?" Sylvia thought to herself that if she stretched herself financially, wouldn't Jane's life plan come to fruition? Didn't she owe this to her daughter?

The therapist identified another theme in Sylvia's automatic internal thoughts: her perceived inadequacies. For example, Sylvia believed that after her first husband died, she neglected her two young children because she was so depressed. She also looked back on her reaction when Jane was being pressured into sex and derided herself for being too passive. Sylvia told Dr. M, "I can't tolerate that I did not protect her. I was not available for her; I allowed her to flounder in school." Sylvia reflexively blamed herself for Jane's current poor decisions and her lack of initiative to improve herself.

Identifying Thought Distortions

Dr. M helped Sylvia identify several types of thought distortions she had. Certainly, Jane was using *all or nothing* thinking. She believed if she didn't stretch herself financially and provide all the money that Jane asked for, then she would be entirely responsible for Jane's financial ruin. Jane would hate her if she failed to provide the loan. Maybe they would never speak again. On the other hand, the loan could allow Jane's boyfriend to finally build a profitable business and put his past behind him. The loan could be the ticket to prosperity for Jane. Maybe the loan would make Jane love her more and the two of them could enjoy spending more time together. This might be her chance to breathe new life into her relationship with Jane. To Sylvia, it was all or nothing. There was no middle ground.

Dr. M encouraged Sylvia to take a step back from the extremes of all or nothing thinking, and said that reframing this thought would yield a more balanced approach. By looking at past patterns of Jane's behavior, Dr. M and Sylvia concluded that the loan might only help Jane temporarily. The loan itself represented a continued practice of Sylvia rescuing Jane from her cycle of need. Why is this loan different from all the other loans that have gone unpaid? Is this approach to getting a loan from her mother really a way to manipulate her? Have other attempts to help Jane actually improved her circumstances or just held her at bay until the next crisis occurs?

By substituting rational alternatives to the premise that the money would make or break Jane, Sylvia was able to decrease her anxiety. While Jane may be angry or disappointed when her mother says no to her the next time, Dr. M reminded her that Jane has been mad before and their relationship still survived. While she might stop talking to Sylvia for a short time, Jane will come back when she is ready.

Sylvia is also demonstrating the distortion of thinking known as *personalization and blame*. She is dumping all her insecurities about her child-rearing into one particularly upsetting request from Jane. She is telling herself that failing to give Jane all the financial and emotional support she required as a child has turned Jane into the woman she is now. Sylvia blames herself for Jane's choices and believes she can remedy a long history of turmoil by helping one more time.

Next Sylvia and Dr. M work to correct this distortion with a rational alternative. Jane is a grown woman. Sylvia must allow Jane to take responsibility for her own decisions. She is not coming to Sylvia for advice, but asking her mother to rescue her after the fact. This is a thankless task. By Sylvia only blaming herself, she is not accounting for how Jane's mood problems and impulsivity have contributed to poor decisions. Furthermore, it is unproductive to use self-blame as an excuse to give in to every request of her adult child, whether valid or not. While Sylvia may have regrets about Jane's upbringing, this does not make Sylvia solely responsible for the future of Jane's boyfriend's business.

Finally, Sylvia is *minimizing* her past attempts to raise Jane as a responsible individual. Instead, she is focusing on the many ways she thinks that she let her child down, while failing to account for all her positive efforts. Correcting this distortion involves enumerating all the ways that she parented effectively in the past. For example, Sylvia had told Jane repeatedly as a child that she loved her and she also had demonstrated affection. Sylvia had tried her best to provide for Jane and her other child generously, even though her finances were sparse. She had worked hard to give her children a good home in a safe neighborhood. She had open communication with their teachers. She attended as many school events as her schedule would allow. She tried to get to know their friends.

When Jane started to have increasing troubles during her teen years, Sylvia took her to counseling, although Jane refused to cooperate. But at least Sylvia had *tried*. Sylvia also knew the value of finishing school and did all she could to help Jane graduate. In retrospect, there may have been other ways Sylvia could have helped her daughter, but this does not mean that she should minimize her many good parenting efforts.

Correcting cognitive distortions becomes a way to examine an upsetting situation from a rational perspective. It does not rely on "positive thinking" or cheerleading. Instead, it is a way to challenge unpleasant emotions. It looks for evidence to support these emotions. Without the evidence, it drives the patient to objectively examine the situation, and correct erroneous feelings with believable facts.

The lessons of cognitive therapy are transportable. The patient may use these techniques outside of therapy to continue to balance her thoughts. The chart on page 176 illustrates common types of thought distortions and offers a structure to substitute more rational alternatives. For example, in one case, the context is that your son just quit his great job at his uncle's information technology company. You may panic and think that he'll never get another job. The thought distortion in this case is catastrophizing, or thinking that whatever is the worst possible thing that could happen *will* happen.

The Behavioral Component of CBT

Dr. M and Sylvia spent a lot of time restructuring Sylvia's thoughts. In addition, they identified behavioral goals to help improve Sylvia's coping capacity and reduce her anxiety. For example, Sylvia wanted to maintain a relationship with her daughter, but she did not want Jane to dictate the terms. They devised three ways that Sylvia could establish appropriate boundaries.

First, because Sylvia dreaded unexpected phone calls and drop-in visits from Jane pleading for money, Sylvia would become proactive in regulating the frequency of the calls and meetings. She would inform Jane that they would speak twice a week at prescribed times with a ten- to fifteen-minute

Thought Distortion Examples

Context	Automatic Thought to Self	Type of Thought Distortion	Better Replacement Thought
My adult child needs money for rent.	I must give my adult child whatever she needs because she is my child. I am responsible for her regardless of my own financial or emotional suffering.	All or Nothing Thinking	It's irrational for me to extend myself if I am unable. I am not responsible for my adult child's failures or her successes. I need to set boundaries for what is reasonable and what is not.
My child just got a neck tattoo right before a family wedding.	My family will be appalled. They will think he is odd or violent. I will be embarrassed when they see him.	Mind Reading	I really don't know what they will think. I am just predicting negative thoughts. Tattoos are not unusual anymore. My relatives will see he is still the sweet kid he always was. No one will pay much attention to it after they see the tattoo for the first time.
My son quit his great job at his uncle's information technology company.	He will never make a living. He is indecisive. Other kids have already forged careers. My son must be irresponsible. He may not find another job. I may have to support him forever.	Catastrophizing	My worst prediction has not happened before. My son has found other jobs soon after quitting in the past. It may take time for him to find his niche, but he manages to land on his feet. I don't need to compare him to my friends' kids. Everyone goes at his own pace.
My child is getting a divorce from a woman I respect and admire.	Why is this happening to him? Why is this happening to me? She did all the right things. She's a good person and has really tried to make it work. It's not fair.	Fallacy of fairness	Life can seem unfair sometimes but it's really not about fairness. Bad things happen to good people. My son has great qualities. It may take awhile but his former wife will rebuild her life and find her happiness.

limit. Secondly, Sylvia would offer to meet Jane once a month for coffee, with a rule that asking for money is not allowed at these meetings. This allows continuance of the relationship, but sets limits to its scope. Finally, Sylvia has decided to give money to Jane only on her birthday and Christmas. She will communicate this to Jane and provide a sum she considers reasonable.

CHANGE OR "RIGHT-SIZE" YOUR EXPECTATIONS

A desirable goal of all therapy is to manage your expectations for your child. Not everyone is born to lead a business or even go to college. Your job as parents is to aim high for your children, but also not lose sight of reality.

Walt, a retired lieutenant general, struggled with shattered hope for his brilliant twenty-five-year-old son. Aaron had developed schizophrenia and in the last few years, his paranoid thoughts and violent behaviors had resulted in two hospitalizations and an inpatient admission for substance abuse. Despite his high intelligence, Aaron dropped out of college and showed no ability to move forward.

Walt said, "His doctor described schizophrenia as a brain disease, so I knew that Aaron was not at fault. But we live in a world where everyone asks about your kid. I hated this type of conversation; I always changed the subject. I didn't know if I was ashamed about Aaron's illness or too tired to lie about it."

The transition to realistic expectations is difficult, and Walt needed time to work this issue out with his wife and therapist. Walt said, "A few years ago, I expected Aaron to be a military officer. Now, I just hope he shows up for his weekly urine drug test at the probation office." Recently, Walt concluded that it would be easier if he changed his response to probing questions about his son. "I just say that he is struggling day to day and all we want is for him to be as happy as he can be. And I leave it at that and just smile if anyone presses me for more details."

Unfulfilled expectations can torment parents, and it is wise to pair your hopes to your adult child's capabilities. Mickey and Kim chose a small college for their son after he struggled in high school. Within a few weeks, it was clear that Peter could not get along with his roommate. He abruptly left school. Mickey and Kim rationalized that maybe a nicer roommate in a new school would help, and they found Peter another college. But at this school, Peter felt too anxious to attend classes and he lasted about a semester.

As their debt mounted and their relationships suffered, Mickey and Kim decided to seek a professional evaluation for Peter, who was diagnosed with both obsessive-compulsive disorder (OCD) and mild autism spectrum disorder. Treatment started, and again Peter enrolled in college, this time a community college close to home. But yet again, it did not take and Peter could not manage. Sometimes people, including your adult children, are not ready for the life choices you hope they will make, and instead, they need to choose another course for themselves. The chart below offers examples of original parental expectations that have been "right-sized" to be realistic.

Right-Sizing Your Expectations

Hopes and Expectations	More Realistic Expectations
Your son should graduate from a good college.	Your son should get his GED.
Your daughter should get a great job.	Your daughter gets any job.
Your adult child should live in a nice house.	Your adult child should have a place to live.
Your son should marry and have children.	Your son will have a positive relationship with someone.
Your daughter should drive a nice car.	Your daughter should have a driver's license that was not suspended.

How do you right-size your expectations for your child? Every family does it differently. Mickey and Kim listened to their family therapist who suggested that they find Peter's strengths rather than revisiting his weaknesses. Peter settled into their small family business, and he organized the company web page and introduced the business to social media. He proudly took the title of Director of Information Technology. Even without a formal degree, both Peter and his parents were gratified with his accomplishments. They also felt much less pressured than in the days when they were trying to fit Peter, a square peg, into the round hole of a college student.

Parents of difficult adult children might cue the example of younger parents who, by a simple twist of fate, give birth to a child with disabilities. "My oldest child Curtis is a natural athlete and a strong student and Jake, my nine-year-old, has Down syndrome," said Emily, a mother in her thirties. "On any given day we might go to Curt's science fair or hear him play violin in the school orchestra. Off in the corner we watch Jake happily playing Angry Birds or enthusiastically engaging an adult, his new best friend, in a deep conversation about his favorite action figure. I get joy from watching both of them."

KEY POINTS IN THIS CHAPTER

- Take care of your physical health and don't ignore serious health conditions you may have, such as hypertension, diabetes, and other major disorders.
- Pay attention to your emotional health as well. If you become depressed or anxious, consider seeing a mental health professional for help.
- Therapy can be very helpful, such as cognitive behavioral therapy (CBT), which teaches individuals to identify irrational thoughts and replace them with realistic thoughts.
- Consider whether your expectations for your child are realistic. If not, then "right-size" them.

Coping with a demanding adult child can be very hard on your relationships with the other people in your life, such as your spouse or partner, your other adult or adolescent children, and family members and friends. That type of coping is the subject of the next chapter.

CHAPTER 10

YOUR RELATIONSHIPS WITH FAMILY AND FRIENDS

My best friend of thirty-nine years said that she was breaking off our friendship. She said that she didn't want to hear about my son's problems anymore because it was just too upsetting to her. I guess I must have said too much. I wish that I had sensed that I was making her uncomfortable and I'm sorry that she did not tell me sooner. This is a very painful loss for me.

When you are enduring the seemingly never-ending ordeal that is your adult child's life, it's difficult to manage other important relationships. Your spouse, partner, children, and friends all may be affected by the behavior of your adult child, either through direct contact with him or indirectly from your responses to him. The divorce rates in these families are high, and far too often, the strain of a troubled adult child destroys second marriages or dooms budding relationships. Siblings witness the unfiltered details; they can't escape the arguing and they might actually be in the direct line of fire. Friendships get the shortest shrift, and keeping secrets—or talking too much about your adult child—may break even strong ties.

One of the challenges of parenting a troubled adult child is to avoid becoming solely defined by this singular relationship. The great struggle is to find balance with other meaningful connections. This chapter focuses on these key relationships and explores case studies of parents who have tried and sometimes succeeded in finding harmony elsewhere in their lives.

COLLATERAL DAMAGE: BLAKE AND ANNE

Each spouse or partner will process the parenting experience differently. This is to be expected. For example, Blake was an avid sportsman, while his wife Anne loved fine art and music, and each respected the other's passion. For many years they were content, but their marriage began to falter when the stress of coping with their only daughter became too overwhelming.

Tanya was the older of their two children. As a teenager, she was diagnosed with oppositional defiant disorder (ODD). In her senior year of high school, Tanya began excessive drinking and she behaved erratically, sometimes nice and sometimes obnoxious, and beyond how other teenagers acted. Then she became pregnant by a random boyfriend. Her mother Anne unsuccessfully objected to Tanya's decision to have an abortion.

Things deteriorated further. Once in college, Tanya did not attend classes and she became involved with a fringe religious movement. Within months, she dropped out of school and found part-time work in a craft store. Blake and Anne tried to get Tanya in treatment, but she rebuffed their outreach. Tanya left the campus and traveled to Toronto with two friends, but soon that support system melted away. She experimented with heroin and became a prostitute to support her growing addiction. Tanya's contact with her parents dropped off, but every phone call to them was news of yet another crisis. It seemed that her only interest in contacting her parents was to ask them for money.

Blake and Anne responded to their daughter's issues very differently. Anne became more focused on Tanya and tried repeatedly to call and visit her. Anne sent her clothes, had food delivered to her apartment, and sent her much more money than Blake had agreed to. Blake felt this was an unwise strategy and asserted that the only way Tanya would right herself was if Ann disengaged. He was certain that the money was going directly into supporting Tanya's addiction.

The arguments between Blake and Anne intensified. Blake claimed that Anne was obsessed about their daughter and was leaving no room for their own relationship. Anne believed that Blake was so angry with her that he withheld any and all affection. Blake no longer complimented her, and he slept in a different bed. For a few years, the couple moved further apart emotionally, with brief respites whenever Tanya showed some progress. But Tanya's gains were never sustained, and Blake and Anne's relationship slowly collapsed. Within four years, the two divorced, disagreeing on almost everything except the fact that the stress of their oldest daughter contributed to their marriage's failure.

Anne decided to talk to a psychologist about her sadness over the divorce and the fact that she still cared for Blake. She told the therapist, "Blake just disappeared. We no longer connected on any level. I felt that I needed to have another life, but I'm sorry we did not make it." Anne rejected the idea that she could have more effectively divided her time and affection between the two parties. "I only did what good mothers do. But he just wanted to wash his hands of first Tanya and then me."

MAKING IT THROUGH: ERIC AND RHONDA

Eric and Rhonda also struggled considerably, but these two had a better outcome than Blake and Anne. Their twenty-eight-year-old son, Kevin, was a combat veteran of Afghanistan, having served three tours. When he returned stateside, his parents grew concerned about his behavior. They noticed that Kevin was losing weight. He was irritable and argumentative. His sleep cycle was erratic.

As the months ticked by, Kevin became even more miserable. He became isolated from his young son and stopped talking to his wife. After a fight over which he was charged with domestic abuse, Eric and Rhonda stepped in and moved Kevin into their house.

Rhonda demonstrated her resourcefulness. She knew that the Veterans Administration had special services for discharged veterans who were suffering from mental health problems. So she contacted the regional VA Medical Center and they reached out to Kevin immediately. In this safe setting, he recounted recurrent flashbacks from an earlier deployment when the military vehicle he was driving had accidentally struck and killed an Afghani teenager who had darted in front of him. Kevin was diagnosed with post-traumatic stress disorder (PTSD), and he applied for disability payments for his service-related psychiatric condition.

The process of determining whether a person qualifies for a disability often takes years, and during this wait Kevin became angry and bitter. Due to his uncontrollable temper, he fought with his wife (whom he still did not live with), and he was unable to hold a job. Eric and Rhonda housed and financially supported Kevin. The issue of whether he would be granted benefits became Kevin's focus, and he acted as if no one or nothing else mattered. His anger was often directed at his parents. Through it all, Eric and Rhonda stayed strong and united. They still showed each other affection and truly listened to each other, even when they did not agree exactly about how they should help their son and his family.

PROTECTING YOUR RELATIONSHIP

In tough times, some parents of adult children make it through and others don't. Of course the specifics of every case are unique, but there are certain principles you can apply to help your relationship:

- Ask each other about feelings.
- Listen and don't prematurely judge what the other person says.
- Summarize what the other person said.
- Make sure your body language matches your words.
- Don't have the same argument over and over.
- Consider possible solutions.

Ask About Feelings

Ask your partner earnestly about feelings. Don't assume that he feels (or should feel) just the same as you and don't put words in his mouth. Avoid framing things negatively. A question like, "You're not worried about him as much as I am, *are* you?" serves no other purpose than putting your spouse on the defensive.

Listen and Don't Prematurely Judge

When your partner tells you how he feels, do your best to withhold judgment. Do not ridicule, argue with, or discredit his sentiments. Instead, put your emotions aside and think about what is being said. What is the underlying emotion and what is the major point? In heated discussions, it's easy to concentrate on what *you* want to say next, rather than to focus on what is being said now by someone else. This probably happens because we can think faster than others can talk. But by doing this, you risk losing their entire message.

This is a skill that Eric and Rhonda mastered. "I can be a pretty cynical person and as a trial lawyer, I argue all day long," said Eric. "Rhonda can take a while to make her point and I have learned to be patient and to wait and listen. I have the ability to verbally cut her off at the knees, but I try not to. I try to listen and validate. Our discussions are so much more productive when I do it this way."

Summarize What Was Said

In a meaningful exchange, it is helpful to summarize what you heard your partner say. If he says, "I'm upset about all the money we've given Sandy. How foolish of us," you might respond with "It sounds like you feel exasperated about the money that we've given Sandy, and you think it's been far too much." In most cases, your partner will appreciate that you are attempting to understand his feelings and to validate them by attempting a summary. Do not derail your efforts by adding, "But you're wrong. I don't agree with you!" You can express your own opinion later on.

If your summary of what was said is not what your partner meant, then ask him to explain again and listen carefully. Regard yourselves as a team and the purpose of this team is to communicate. Communication involves listening and talking.

Make Sure Your Body Language Matches Your Words

Your body language counts every bit as much as your words. If you say you're happy but you're grimacing with anger, then it's clear you're not being truthful about your feelings. If you say you accept what's going on, but you are standing with arms akimbo on both hips, you are not accepting of the situation. How do you know what your body language shows, since you cannot see yourself? Here's one quick way to know: Do your feelings match the words you are expressing? If not, your body language will give you away. Notice your stance and whether (or not) you are tension-filled. Become more aware of yourself.

If you think you are being perfectly reasonable, go look at yourself in the mirror and observe your face. Does this face communicate a willingness to listen? Or is it an angry face that wants to have its own way?

Abby and Hal have a thirty-year-old son who is constantly in trouble. He was recently placed on probation for shoplifting and they both know that another infraction will likely lead to a prison sentence. The couple disagrees on nearly all aspects of how to respond to their son's behavior. In their most recent battle, they argued about whether to spend thousands of dollars for a private attorney to defend their son. Abby wants to hire a lawyer, but Hal does not.

Abby explained, "It's funny, but we can argue and disagree strongly but if he is looking into my eyes, things are better." The consequence of not being in control of your body language is immediate. "When he gives me partial attention or he walks away while we are talking, I get enraged and then I say desperate and mean things. He gets offended and then we start arguing about the fair way to argue. We lose the original point of the discussion."

Don't Repeat the Same Argument Again and Again

Athletes have muscle memory. If a figure skater performs a jump over and over, it eventually becomes a reflex. Years later, she can still repeat the maneuver without practice. Behaviors follow a similar pattern. Seasoned spouses usually know how their partners will react to a particular event.

Arlene and Michael's twenty-one-year-old son lives with them. Adam has mild autism spectrum disorder (formerly known as Asperger's) and ADHD, and on those days that he does not take his medication, he can barely get out of bed. But when he's on medication, Kevin goes to community college and works part-time at the supermarket.

The battle lines on this issue were established years ago. Arlene feels that it is Adam's responsibility to take his own medications, and says, "He is an adult and I cannot do everything for him."

But Michael counters, "Unless we give the medication to him, his day never starts. It is true he is an adult and we can't live his life for him. But if he cannot do this one essential act of taking his daily medication, all that he has accomplished vanishes. So we must give him his medications so that he actually takes them."

And so it goes. Virtually every day the couple has the same argument. At a recent meeting, their longtime counselor noted, "You were arguing about this on your son's first day of tenth grade and his first day of college." Arlene and Michael looked at each other, nodded in agreement, and laughed. Michael said, "Yes, we have had one argument a thousand different times and each time it's like we are having it for the very first time." Avoid this mistake. Agree to disagree.

In this case, Arlene decided to back off and let Michael give their son his medications every day. Harmony was restored.

Consider Possible Solutions

As you commit yourself to improving communications with your spouse, you can focus on maintaining your momentum. Some couples decide that they need a defined hour each week to discuss their adult child. Beyond that predetermined hour, they make a rule not to broach the subject. Without the rule, the burden can bleed over into all other activities you share with your spouse.

Brainstorm ideas about how best to set aside time to resume activities that you enjoyed together in the past and that you've dropped since your family problems began. Maybe you used to ride bikes, go to the movies, or talk about politics. You deserve some alone time together. During this time, turn your cell phone off and don't log into your e-mail.

THE CENTRALITY OF INTIMACY

Maintaining a close personal relationship with a partner is central to the survival of a relationship. It enhances both people as well as their importance as a couple, even when the unthinkable happens.

After a long struggle with bipolar disorder, Brian shot himself a week after his twenty-sixth birthday. He died from his injuries a month later. His parents Alex and Laurie spent the next year in deep mourning. A year after his death, Alex, a professional artist, began a series of ceramics to memorialize his son.

"It was then that I started to wake up. Brian was gone but we were still here and we still had to live. My art is a way to make sense of my loss," says Alex.

But Laurie could not follow Alex's lead. Her mourning turned into depression. She had little interest in Alex's new project, and he was increasingly frustrated by Laurie's isolation. Bitterness now flowed into their stream of grief.

In a counseling session, Alex lamented their loss of intimacy. "I need my wife and I can't live my life without sex. You are withholding something very important to me."

"I am not withholding," Laurie protested. "It is important to me too. We have been making love for thirty years and it always meant joy and abandon. I just can't escape my own troubling thoughts anymore."

"You are the mother of my child and the object of my desire," Alex replied, "Not one or the other, but both. You will always be that to me."

With that exchange, the couple went home and made love. At their next session, Arlene reflected on their honest exchange and the progress they had made. "I realized that sex with my husband gave me the few moments of escape that I need. Sex exhilarated me when we were younger, but now it heals both of us."

Any honest therapist will concede that epiphanies rarely occur in a therapy session. This was an exception.

Understanding Her Husband Helped

To people on the outside looking in, the O'Conners had it all. Their family was intact and both Linda and Devon had successful careers. Devon was a major fundraiser for the local hospital and an executive for a multinational manufacturing company. He was a personable and effective executive and everyone expected that he would be promoted even higher. Linda was a successful hand surgeon. Their two sons were poised and sociable and had no reservations about driving their late model cars (compliments of their parents) all over town.

Despite these outward trappings, Devon endlessly clashed with his twenty-seven-year-old son Travis, who had been treated for severe ADHD for years. Devon considered Travis's college major, acting, to be "a joke" and viewed his son's tepid GPA as reflecting minimal effort. Devon was also dismayed that his son put forth no effort to secure a reasonable job. He was upset when Travis got his third speeding ticket and was livid when he failed to show up for a charity fundraiser that the family sponsored each year.

Linda was not thrilled with her son either, but she could do nothing to ratchet down the tension. Devon's anger at his son permeated the family and despite their harmonious public image, the family was in turmoil.

Finally, Linda was exasperated and she came for help. She and her therapist spoke about her husband's background. Devon was born into a successful family. His father was a famous engineer who had many patents to his name. His mother served on several of the local philanthropic organizations. Devon's parents emphasized the importance of hard work and public sacrifice. The family creed was service to others. Linda had known all these facts before, but somehow discussing it aloud with the therapist gave it new meaning.

Linda returned to her therapist the next week to further discuss the issue. "The other night after he had another argument with Travis, I approached my husband to talk. I did not admonish him as I usually do—I just listened. We talked about his beliefs and his hopes for our children. Devon knows that ADHD explains many of Travis's behaviors. Still he feels that we spoiled Travis and we are responsible for making him lazy. Life has dealt us a good hand but he can't get over that his own son, who has been given so much, gives back so little."

Linda processed the conversation a bit more, "My husband was embarrassed to admit that he just expected his son to be more like him. Now I understand that when Devon screams, he is blaming himself as much as Travis."

THINKING ABOUT YOUR OTHER CHILDREN

Edward first displayed signs of bipolar disorder by age nine. He had a flash temper and wild mood swings. At times, Edward was convinced that he was being treated unfairly by his family and during these times of paranoia, there was no reasoning with him. He frequently resisted treatment, and once off the medications, he was irritable, demanding, and highly unpredictable.

Edward's younger sister Rory was often present during his rage attacks. Over the years she watched him punch the walls and kick the garage door. At one time or another, he assaulted each family member, once fracturing his sister's wrist. At his worst, Edward threatened to kill his parents and doctors. The threats faded after psychiatric hospitalizations and when he was stabilized on medications.

Rory never was fully comforted. These threats became the substance of her nightmares. She thought about them constantly. When she went to summer camp as a ten-year-old, she was preoccupied with her parents' safety and insisted on daily contact with them. She was convinced that her parents were in peril years later, when she left for college.

Rory's concerns about her brother were not limited to the family's safety. When they were in school together, Edward had a notorious reputation because of his behavior and Rory was deeply embarrassed to be associated with him. She refused to invite friends to her home when he was there. She accused her parents of spending all their time with Edward and neglecting her accomplishments. She was reticent to discuss with her parents the shame she felt about Edward.

Rory's parents redoubled their efforts with her. They traveled to all of her soccer games and made extra efforts to welcome her friends. They made certain to appreciate Rory's academic accomplishments and tried to avoid letting their angst over Edward diminish their pride in her. Most importantly to Rory they acknowledged her fears about the threat that Edward posed. By and large the efforts worked and the family, strained by their circumstances, remained close.

By their early twenties Edward and Rory were on different trajectories. Rory built her professional life, married, and moved to Manhattan.

Edward continued to make unwise choices and have bursts of unpredictable behavior. He was unable to keep a job and retreated to his parents' basement.

The week after Rory's twenty-fifth birthday, her mother was diagnosed with breast cancer. Rory's fears quickly reconstituted. "My mother is pretty sick, but I still think Edward is a bigger threat to her," she said to her husband. "I fear that I will be left caring for him when they can't do it anymore." No other family members lived nearby, and nobody else could step in if her parents became ill or died. Rory feared that the brother who had tormented her throughout her youth would be the albatross of her adult life.

At the urging of her husband, Rory approached her parents. As they did when she was a child, they listened. They agreed that leaving her the responsibility of Edward was too great. Her mother's breast cancer diagnosis was devastating, but it forced the family to plan their future.

Until this time, Edward had been treated by private doctors, but Edward agreed to enroll in the community mental health system in order

SIBLINGS OF SCHIZOPHRENICS

How does a healthy family member feel about his mentally ill sibling? A study published in the *Israel Journal of Psychiatry and Related Sciences* posed this question, and the answer is: Not good. The study compared fifty-two individuals whose siblings had schizophrenia to forty-eight controls whose siblings were not affected.

The researchers found that the siblings of the mentally ill had more intensely negative feelings and a higher level of burden than the control group. This group reported feeling less closeness with their siblings and more shame about them. Mercy be to all who suffer from schizophrenia; there are very few other illnesses that cause such prolonged and perpetual human suffering. This research, however, identified siblings as "secondary victims" of schizophrenia. Like all family members of troubled adults, they need to be supported with education about mental illness. Therapy can provide a healthy outlet to deal with feelings of stigma and shame.

to qualify for a housing program and other wrap-around services for the chronically mentally ill. His parents also consulted an attorney, and decided that to minimize the possibility that Edward would squander any money left to him, Rory would be the executor of their estate. Although the family was not wealthy, they established a small trust fund for Edward to ensure him a small long-term income. To unburden Rory, they also set aside funds for a legal guardian to administer Edward's assets. Taken together, all these actions strengthened the family's bond.

Your Other Children Know What's Going On— And May Not Like It

When one family member presents a major problem for you, whether it is mental illness, substance abuse, or another issue, you generally spend time and resources on that person. It also means that you are spending *less* time thinking about and worrying about your other children. You probably are spending less money on them as well. Healthy siblings undoubtedly can feel shortchanged and less valued than their "problem" brother or sister.

A corollary issue is that your other adult children may develop a sense of entitlement. After all, they may have heard you complain about the thousands of dollars you spent on your mentally ill child. They may ask, "When is it my turn?"

Parents will need to consider various scenarios. What if the mentally healthy child needs a down payment for a new car? Can you afford to turn him down? What if he invites you to visit him for a week in another state— should you defer because you're worried about what will happen if you leave your troubled adult child behind? Or should you leave against your better judgment? Does one child get everything, and the other children receive nothing? Parents have struggled with this fairness issue forever.

Remember that none of your adult children is automatically entitled to your time or your money. Even if you give one adult child an inordinate amount of money (which you now regret because she just used it to buy drugs rather than pay her court fines), the fact is that you did give her that money. It's gone and you can't undo your action. But that does not mean that you should repeat your overspending mistakes with another child. Money does not automatically equal love and giving one child more money does not mean that you love him best. This is a point you can share forcefully with your other children.

FRIENDS AND FAMILY

Graham and Meg raised three children. Their oldest child was a design engineer for General Motors and their youngest child was a respected teacher and rugby coach. Their middle child, however, always was in trouble. Mitchell's diagnosis was unclear but Graham and Meg felt that he matched the profile for antisocial personality disorder. He barely graduated from high school and had gone through five jobs in six years. Mitchell had three children from two different women and he never earned enough money to make any child support payments. Graham and Meg were mortified when the local paper featured him in an article about deadbeat dads.

Graham was forthright about how the ordeal impacted his relationship with his friends and the community, and said, "I have a hard time enjoying the happy times of my friends." Recently he scheduled a travel conflict so he would have an excuse to miss a friend's family wedding. Graham realized that Mitchell's failure revealed his own competitiveness. His son was losing at the game of life, and it embarrassed him.

Meg understood her husband's feelings. "Our other children and grandchildren are doing well, but Mitchell's problems cast a long shadow." Unlike her husband, Meg was able to share in her friends' happy times, but she has also become increasingly intolerant of their careless comments. She addressed the issue of friends at a Families Anonymous Meeting and was surprised how strongly it resonated with the other parents of troubled adult children. The group exchanged their most frustrating encounters with their well-intentioned friends. Group members noted that sometimes friends make well-meant but aggravating statements, such as:

- You only get problems you can handle.
- You should never see your child again.
- Too many people are on psychiatric drugs.

You Only Get Problems You Can Handle

Mary reported, "I will scream if someone else tells me that God only gives people the problems that they can handle. This is exasperating to hear, because I am falling apart. I may run down the street screaming if the situation gets any worse. And this other person seems to be saying that I *should* handle it because I can. Well, how does he or anyone else know that?" Another couple laughed at the cross-cultural popularity of the statement, and said that when they lived in California, they were told that it was karma that gives you what you can handle. "We decided not to engage in this type of conversation. It served no purpose."

You Should Never See Your Child Again

Helen's son was addicted to methamphetamine. Helen says, "Whenever we get a chance to help him, we do. Usually he is clean for a couple of months, then he goes back to using." She continues, "My good friend has been vaguely aware of our problems for years and I was hurt when she told me to let go and cut all ties with my son." Helen believes that her friend is entitled to her opinion, but she didn't ask for one and she doesn't agree with her friend. Helen reflected, "Maybe we are helping our son—maybe we are enabling him, but she does not have the full story, she is not an expert, and she does not have a vote in this."

Too Many People Are on Psychiatric Drugs

Paul, Mary's husband, recalled attending a church service where the visiting pastor blamed psychiatric medications for many of society's difficulties. In a follow-up discussion, Paul's cousin echoed the theme of too many people taking psychiatric medications. He had read an article about someone who became suicidal on antidepressant medications. "My cousin said that medications were the cause of our daughter's problems. I could not contain myself. I told him that it was like saying that drinking water makes you thirsty. These people mix up the problem and the solution."

Paul continued, "Before I got too mad, I remembered that my interest is not in defending the entire universe of people who take psychiatric medications. My focus is on my adult child alone. And he needs medications to help him."

FINDING BALANCE

The stress of dealing with an intractable problem impacts a parent's relationship to his spouse, his family, and friends. It is an ongoing struggle to find a balance where the dedication to your child does not snuff out your connections to others. Jerry takes her two golden retrievers to the local park each morning and relaxes with other owners as their dogs run. It is not always easy to relax. Her puppy Wilson runs with the pack and listens to commands. In contrast four-year-old retriever Clyde darts into the woods and sometimes onto the street, a habit that has not been broken by the city's best dog trainers.

Jerry returned home and fumed to her husband one morning. "We had a new guy in the group today. He said that dogs always run away for a reason. They want to be free of their owner. Well if he is right, why is Wilson always at my side?" She decided not to be angry with the new guy.

You can't always control your dogs or your children. One of the essential truths of coping with troubled children is learning the limitations of parenting. Later you seek to locate that precarious balance where your dedication to your children does not wipe out your connection to others.

KEY POINTS IN THIS CHAPTER

- Don't forget that as you suffer with the issues your adult child is facing, your spouse or partner is also suffering. Try to keep in touch with each other's feelings and act collaboratively.

- Your other children are affected by your adult child as well as by your reactions. Try to keep them in the loop about what is going on and also have conversations with them about their own problems. The "good" children need attention too.

- Avoid repeated battles with your partners on the same issues. Agree to disagree.

- Many people will say annoying things to you, but try to take it in stride. There's a plethora of ignorance about adult children with issues.

The next chapter covers strategies that may help you and your adult child resolve some (but probably not all) of the serious problems that your child faces.

CHAPTER 11

SETTING LIMITS: WHAT YOU CAN OR CAN'T DO

I'm an accountant, so I keep track of all my expenses. I have spent close to $50,000 buying my daughter used cars when she runs a current car into the ground, and paying her rent, utility bills, and so forth. I'm okay now financially, but cannot give her any more without jeopardizing myself. I cannot let her ruin me financially. It's really up to her now.

Laurie was in her third year of college at a large Midwestern university when the voices in her head started. At first she tried to drown them out by turning up the volume on her iPod. Then Laurie soon noticed that crowds made the voices much louder, so she stopped going to lectures. Her roommates also noticed that Laurie had changed. She had become angry and reclusive, and she slept most of the day, leaving the apartment at odd times.

Late in the semester Renee received a phone call from the campus police. Laurie had been found sleeping in the local cemetery, and she was brought to the university hospital to treat an unexplained gash to her forehead. Upon hearing the news, Renee rushed to the hospital. Her relief that her daughter was safe was tempered by the subsequent news from the ER doctor. Laurie was two months pregnant.

In another case, Peter started drinking heavily in high school. As his sister left for college and then a job and his brother excelled in professional hockey, Peter spent the next decade moving from job to job, from girlfriend A to girlfriend B, and so on. His parents knew that he was creative, but Peter shared none of their enthusiasm for using his artistic talents. By age nineteen, he had been arrested twice for drunk driving. By age twenty-one, Peter had already served six months in jail for petty larceny. As a condition of his release, he reluctantly agreed to participate in a substance treatment program. But Peter's sobriety did not last long.

HOPES VERSUS REALITIES

All parents hope that their dependent children will flourish into independent adults. But the Rolling Stones said it best, "You can't always get what you want." Being a good parent doesn't mean that you will be rewarded with an easy child to raise.

Laurie's sudden decline represents the opening salvo in a struggle with chronic paranoid schizophrenia. The vignette of Peter's life is one of countless episodes of bad judgment and irresponsible behavior. The parents of mentally ill or otherwise debilitated adult children are left to synthesize a plan to cope with the ongoing dependency. At a time in their lives when they expected to see their children soar, they are forced to scrape them up off the floor.

Parents of adult children with serious issues think and worry about the long haul. How will my adult child be cared for? How do I pay for her needs? How far do I go to help him without hurting him? This chapter attempts to address these elemental questions.

Among the first realizations is that so little is under parental control. Your adult child, however vulnerable or self-defeating he may be, is still an adult and he makes the final decisions about his life. For example, Peter was offered all the perks of affluence, from the best schools to the nicest clothes, and when he needed it, the best mental health treatment. To his parents' frustration, however, he never was resourceful enough to use these advantages.

Renee recalls the devastation of learning of her daughter's mental illness right after the pregnancy was discovered. Immediately, Renee felt that she had to make decisive moves. She brought Laurie home to live and Renee read about schizophrenia, the diagnosis that Laurie had been given. Also Renee contacted Families Anonymous, a support group for families battling mental illness. Renee also helped Laurie find a caring psychiatrist. Another step that Laurie could have taken was to take a free twelve-week course on mental illness with the National Alliance for Mental Illness (NAMI). The course is called "Family to Family Education Program." For more information, go to nami.org/template.cfm?Section=Family-to-Family&lstid=751.

Parents of troubled adult children often worry about ensuring their child has health care should they become ill. Laurie is no longer a student. Her family was grateful to learn that under the federal Affordable Care Act, adult children are allowed to stay on their parents' insurance until age twenty-six.

Renee decided to help her daughter pursue Supplemental Security Insurance (SSI). Medicaid benefits are automatic for individuals who receive SSI payments.

Yet as strongly as Renee willed her daughter to get all better, Laurie's progress was slow. Laurie's hallucinations continued and her bizarre behavior grew worse. She also refused to get any obstetrical care throughout her pregnancy. Renee said, "I felt alone and overmatched. I was making most of the decisions, but I could not lose the fact that Laurie had sovereign rights. I thought she should have an abortion, but doctors were reluctant to perform the procedure on a psychotic woman." Also, Laurie was ambivalent herself about having an abortion.

Laurie received antipsychotic medications from her psychiatrist, who believed that the risk for extreme and self-destructive behavior from Laurie was greater than the risk of antipsychotics for a pregnant woman. Fortunately, the baby was born healthy and was later adopted by relatives who were both eager and able to raise a child and who were not worried about a possible genetic risk for mental illness that the child might have inherited.

DEMANDING CERTAIN THINGS, INCLUDING TREATMENT

So little is under a parent's control that you must maximize whatever influence you have. Previous chapters stressed the importance of treatment, and the same message applies to Laurie and Peter. Yet sometimes even the best treatment has its limitations. "Once Laurie started taking Clozaril, the voices went away, but she was still not the same person," said Renee. "Our sweet teenager had turned into a distant and unemotional young adult. She didn't like the side effects of gaining weight or being tired. Still I insisted that she take her medications and she did. She knew that there was no other acceptable way."

In uncontrolled situations, parents need to do all that can be done. Peter's parents, Craig and Nora, negotiated a common understanding with their recalcitrant son. Like many individuals with antisocial personality disorder, Peter did not pursue treatment because he saw little reason to change. Nora said, "We knew that Peter's alcohol craving went way down when he took Campral. We were determined to get through his two years of probation without an ugly episode." They made a simple agreement: If Peter would take his medications that week, then his parents would fill his car with gas. "It somehow actually worked," said Nora.

FINDING BALANCE

It is impossible to make it through life without getting rained on, but there are many different degrees of saturation. You may listen to your neighbors or coworkers complain about minor inconveniences or a temporary money crunch, but you know (although you keep the thought to yourself) that many of their issues are minor and will soon resolve themselves. In contrast, the parents of chronically ill children live their anxiety every day and often have little hope of relief. Each day brings new problems, which may grow more complicated with time.

Work with your adult child so that you and she can try to make solid decisions that are both good for your child and also fair to other family members. This is by no means an easy road to navigate.

Adopting a Hard-Line Approach

Jenny was a person who pushed everyone to the limits. She was adopted at age three and her parents Tanya and Joe, approaching age forty at the time of the adoption, never could keep up with Jenny. She exerted little effort in middle school and in high school Jenny assumed the position of chairperson of the mean girls. Jenny drank on weekends, and spent most of her time finding and then dropping boyfriends and excluding other girls from any social recognition. By her senior year, both the school administration and her fellow students knew of her malicious ways. Jenny was transferred to an alternative high school and barely graduated.

Many of Jenny's former classmates, to whom she had been so malignant, went on to college, the military, or a family business. Jenny had few options and she withered most of them away. She started waitressing but was found stealing from the cash register and was fired. Her roommate, with whom she had been sharing an apartment, moved out after six months, leaving Jenny with a large debt. (She had neglected to have the friend co-sign the rental agreement and consequently Jenny had complete liability.) Jenny turned to her parents to cover the loss, and they did so.

Over the next five years, Jenny lived with three consecutive boyfriends, and worked three or four part-time jobs. As was the case through most of her life, Tanya and Joe had little influence on their daughter. After years of this chaos, Tanya remarked, "It's sad that her only accomplishment so far is that she has not become pregnant."

When Jenny was twenty-four, she asked to move home and Tanya and Joe reluctantly agreed. They were right to be reluctant. For most of the next two years, Jenny did not work and she regularly slept until noon. She would dress provocatively and party late into the night with no regard for her parents or younger siblings' schedule. When Tanya and Joe discovered that some expensive jewelry was missing, they did not know whether to suspect Jenny or one of the many random people she had brought into their home.

"At that point, I was done," said Tanya, "I was at the limit. We told Jenny that she had to leave. We could not be a part of her life anymore. It hurt us too much to watch her self-destruct, and we did not think we were helping her in any way. We had to try something new."

Jenny resisted leaving home. However, soon she found a new boyfriend to move in with, but this relationship lasted only a few weeks. She called her parents asking for another try. "No" was the unified answer. Tanya said, "We told Jenny, yes, you will have to go to the homeless shelter if you have nowhere else to sleep. And no, we will not give you any more money." The message was clear. Jenny had to show some progress before her parents would consider rescuing her once again.

Six months passed with little contact between the parents and their daughter. Tanya and Joe worried constantly about Jenny's well-being.

Every time he put his head on the pillow at night, Joe wondered if Jenny was in a safe place. At times, Joe was critical of his wife's hard line, but they agreed to not relent from their position.

They did not know that Jenny had finally connected with their message. At the woman's shelter, Jenny noticed a posting for work in a United Way program. The head of the program, a gentle local pastor, liked Jenny and offered her a job distributing meals to poor families. Jenny became part of his organization and she quickly excelled. She learned the importance of teamwork and personal responsibility. Jenny stopped using her sexuality to manipulate people and instead she displayed her gregarious personality to spur more donations.

Several years later, Jenny was asked to lead the local program, and the family celebrated Jenny's thirtieth birthday together. She was now functioning well. The only question is whether her transformation was due to the passage of time or her parents' dramatic decision to back off and force her to mature. But the most important issue for them was the outcome: a happier and more successful Jenny.

Working the Deal with Peter: A Softer Approach

Many parents can swap stories about their adult child's money mismanagement, but not all have Tanya and Joe's firm resolve. Peter's father Craig shared the following: "We could not control Peter's spending. He was great at getting credit cards and spending them to the limit. I am a businessman, so I really believe in paying your debts. I paid his bills at first because I thought it was the right thing to do."

His wife Nora was angry at her son and she was even angrier at her husband. She accused Craig of enabling Peter by covering for him all the time. Craig said, "My wife told me that if Peter had carte blanche, then he would never take any responsibility. I realized that this is true and that I gave him money to avert my own emotional pain that I felt when my son was deprived." Craig had the conflicted emotions of being angry at Peter's poor choices and sad that those choices left his son with so little.

In deference to Nora, Craig tried a harder line. He said, "We then went through a period where we paid for nothing. This was not so wonderful either. When he had no money, Peter did nothing and he just spent all his time in the basement. We were unhappy that he was always around." The couple found no happiness with either indulging or depriving their son.

After several months of a cold war with his wife, Craig developed a guiding principle. "I decided to pay for things for Peter if they are in our best interests too." As an example, Craig decided to pay for Peter's car insurance, rationalizing that if his son had no transportation, then he could not get a job.

"I paid for basic coverage for his cell phone so that his work could reach him and I could contact him anytime I wanted," said Craig, adding, "But I refused to get him the newest smartphone with the deluxe data package." This pragmatic compromise worked for Craig and Nora.

To further improve their credibility, Craig and Nora insisted that all obligations be clarified. To avoid misunderstandings, a laminated list of weekly tasks and other expectations for Peter is taped to the refrigerator. They also demand he contribute to solving his own financial problems. For example, three years ago, Peter had an unpaid $20,000 credit card.

Nora said, "We agreed to pay half of the bill provided that he would make his contribution without disruption. We never missed a week and never let him free of his portion even at Christmas. He knew that this agreement was inviolable. Last week we paid it off."

FINANCIAL PLANNING

Don was diagnosed with mild autism spectrum disorder early in middle school. The public school district provided Don with many resources. His principal put together an Individualized Educational Plan (IEP) that followed Don through high school. Don had access to a resource room and he participated in a tailored curriculum. He was assigned a teacher's aide and also received regular psychological counseling. Don had difficulty making friends, but a kind teacher found him a place on the computer robotics team.

Don was handed a diploma at graduation but in exchange, he and his family gave up the beneficial school services. At that time, there was little community support for young adults with debilitating social anxiety and an awkward interpersonal style. In the depths of the last recession, Don was unable to find a job. He spent his days playing video games, and the bulk of his social contacts were virtual, such as fellow World of Warcraft players whom he had never met.

After several years of this pattern, it became clear that Don was not making progress. His family met to share their mutual concerns. His mother, a widow recently diagnosed with ovarian cancer, worried about who would care for Don in the event that her illness progressed. Don's two sisters had similar concerns. Neither sister was prepared to bring Don into their home, and both worried about how to support Don and who would make decisions for him.

The meeting spurred the family into action. Don's sister contacted Friendship Circle, a nonprofit Michigan-based organization that helps individuals with special needs. Many similar organizations have taken root throughout the country, and in some states, they have helped secure legislation mandating that insurance companies cover services for this population. The family was assigned a professional advocate who found Don a workshop program for socialization to prepare for a job. The family helped Don apply for Supplemental Security Income (SSI) and state Medicaid.

As importantly, the family mustered the courage to talk about their finances. The daughters knew that after their father's sudden death, his estate had been transferred to their mother. They worried that when their mother died, Don would be left a third of the estate and both sisters feared that he would squander the money that he needed to last him a lifetime.

Guided by the family advocate, their mother agreed to hire a probate attorney who set up a living trust that ensured Don a monthly income but never gave him total control of all the funds. Both of Don's sisters lived out of town and they were relieved that a legal guardian would be appointed to manage their brother's daily affairs. The family rested more comfortably knowing that their money was being professionally invested and that Don would be left well positioned.

BREAKING DOWN PROBLEMS

There are many ways that adult children can break your heart. Most heartbreak results from bad decisions. Your children may spend money impulsively, pursue poisonous relationships, or get into major legal binds. At each bruising turn, your child grows more frustrated as your faith in him erodes.

There are some basic rules to help your child make good decisions. These rules are fundamental for the parents of young children, but they also need to be reinforced in adult children who are intellectually limited or emotionally immature. These rules are most crucially needed by individuals with substance abuse problems or antisocial personality disorder, as those with these conditions often teeter on the precipice of disaster. Their general disregard for methodical approaches to problem solving makes implementing the rules quite tricky, yet their ongoing turmoil often demands your input.

Ask Basic Who, What, When, Where, Why, and How Much Questions

Begin by explaining that you will try to help by exploring your child's major problems in a structured way. Sometimes by talking through the elements of a troubling situation, a previously ignored solution suddenly presents itself. This process, used by journalists trying to grasp the basic elements of a story, can be productive because the child has previously resisted thinking about the issue or is too overwhelmed by its magnitude.

Many times individuals with antisocial personality disorder understand that they have entered a problematic quicksand, but they are too impatient to explain all the details to you. Be clear to her that helping with her issues does not mean that you intend to heroically rescue her from responsibility. Your goal is to develop a structure for her to pay her bills, but it is not an offer for you to do it for her.

Whatever the problem, you can learn more by asking your adult child some key questions. Find out *who* is the person in the power position of the problem? Is it the boss, the bank, the landlord, the police? Then ask *what* the problem is, as far as your child knows. Will the electricity be cut off because a bill was not paid? Did a failed drug test trigger a violation of their probation?

When are the results of the problem going to occur? Will the consequence occur today, tomorrow, or next month? In many cases, there is a specific date by which some action must be taken. The "whens" are often ignored, yet these details are very important. Many complications can be avoided simply by paying a bill on time or by showing up for court on the right date.

Clarify *where* the event will happen. Is your child being arraigned at the courthouse? Is a state official coming to her house to investigate? And *why* is it happening? Yes, the eviction process may be starting because a bill wasn't paid, but you may learn that your child was temporarily unable to work. This provides the *why* explanation.

Jackie's son was recently released from prison, and he got a job selling merchandise at the baseball stadium. Jackie said, "He actually did well for a few months but there were several rainouts and he earned nothing for a while. The landlord was sympathetic when Jackie explained this to his landlord. Crisis avoided . . . for now." Some businesses will extend the grace period of payment at least a few days if the individual calls and explains the problem, asking (politely!) for extra time.

You will also need to determine *how much* it will cost to resolve the problem. For example, if your child owes five hundred dollars and she cannot pay it at once, can she make a partial payment with a guarantee that the balance will be paid by a certain date? Again, if your child could not pay the bill because she was very sick or in the hospital, there is nothing lost in asking for a reprieve. The favor should be paired with proof (e.g., a doctor's note) to avoid the suspicions that are naturally generated when an excuse is offered.

Once the scope of the problem is understood, you and your adult child are in a better position to work on a solution.

Prioritizing Problems

Problem solving also requires some triage, so it is helpful to have your child list her ten most serious problems. Then have her prioritize these problems from the most pressing one (or the one with the most imme-diate consequences) to the least important issue. The plan is to work together on Problem Number One first, and then knock each one off in appropriate order.

If you think that your child has misjudged her list, then discuss it in a positive fashion. For example, it might be disconcerting to you if she gives the highest priority to her unpaid bill with the storage unit where she's keeping her furniture, over the priority for her unpaid rent. If so, then ask her, and in a noncondescending manner, what is more concerning to you, having your old furniture confiscated or not having a roof over your head? She may not like the idea of losing her furniture, but the direct question forces a qualitative analysis of her priorities.

If your child continues to insist that the payment for the storage unit is her most pressing problem, then move on to the next issue rather than arguing over this issue. As you continue to go through the list, she may realize herself that her priorities should change. Do not easily succumb to offering your home, yet again, as a way out for her. She is an adult and needs to learn to live in the outside world, albeit belatedly.

What Has He Already Tried?

You also need to ask your adult child if he has had this problem before and what he did then to resolve the issue. He may surprise you and may have already tried to work something out. If so, you need to know what he offered and how the person in power responded. Said Lisa about her son Rick, age thirty-one, "We spent an hour talking about his latest conundrum when Rick told me that last year his landlord allowed him to paint the hall-ways in exchange for the full rent. I wanted to scream at him, 'Why didn't you tell me that earlier?' But I resisted." The more methodically your child can provide you the information and the calmer you are when you receive it (no matter how maddening the response may sometimes be), then the easier it should be for the two of you to work through the issues.

You should also ask your adult child to think of the landlord as a per-son who should be treated with politeness and fairness. Try to guide your child away from demonizing those to whom they owe money. Portray the landlord as a businessman who needs the rent money to pay his employees, and not as an evil exploiter not worthy of respect. In another example, if your adult child speaks disrespectfully about his probation officer, you should recast the officer as an average person who is enforcing the county policy, and not a personal enemy. Your child may not be empathetic by nature, but there is nothing to be gained if he hears you are also denigrating his foils.

You may be able to find other solutions for your child to try. In general, however, it is best that your child use your ideas as his own and then for you to back off. Be mindful that unless you let *him* implement the solution, nothing is gained. For example, if you communicate with the landlord directly, then *you* will be perceived as the solution by both your child and the landlord. If problems occur downstream the landlord will bypass your child and contact you directly for a resolution.

Brainstorming Solutions

Have a brainstorming session in which you and your child discuss possible solutions to the current issue. It's okay if the ideas are silly. Even crazy ideas may be valuable because they may trigger thoughts of possible remedies to the problem. Write them all down and discuss all the strategies together. Your adult child may brainstorm that she loves her house and wishes she could buy it. Her sentiment should be shared with the landlord as he too probably loves the property and at least on this account, he and your daughter share common ground.

Obviously this is not a resolution; if she can't make the rent, she has little chance of making the down payment. Not all the ideas will be winners, but the process of brainstorming is a fundamental means to resourceful thinking and should be encouraged.

A Willingness to Ask for Help

Many communities have social services available for those in need. Religious organizations and governmental agencies may provide short-term housing. Many of these groups sponsor or can refer your child to free health clinics whose mission is to serve the indigent. Most states offer generous benefits to pregnant mothers and their children through state Medicaid. Children born to poor mothers also have access to the Women, Infants and Children (WIC) program and other nutritional programs (nutrition .gov/food-assistance-programs/wic-women-infants-and-children).

But your child needs to be able to ask for help. When Monica called her daughter who lived a thousand miles away, Carla complained that she had no food in her kitchen. Typically this is when Carla would ask for money, as she had done countless times before. This time Monica was prepared to offer a more constructive response. She encouraged Carla to apply for Food Stamps. In the short run, suggested Monica, Carla should visit the local Salvation Army and ask for food. Carla responded with horror, and said, "Mom! Those places are for *poor* people! I'm not going there." Monica assured her daughter that she was not too good to ask for help.

Is Monica's decision not to send her daughter money an example of shifting a family's responsibility to a charity or government? To some degree that is true. Still these social service agencies exist to help the downtrodden. Once your child reaches out to them for food or shelter, most agencies will work to reinforce behaviors that promote independence.

Why Is It Different This Time?

Even after you insist that your child go through the process of brainstorming and problem solving, you might, once again, decide that there is no other alternative but for you to intervene and assume the financial and emotional burden. If at the end of the process you are again paying the bill, why even go through the painstaking process?

For several reasons. First, your child should be aware that he needs to reciprocate. If you are good enough to pay part of his rent, he should clean out the messy garage. If you take care of her children because she has not planned well, she must agree to paint the bedroom.

More importantly, your adult child must understand that his behavior is unacceptable, and although you are responding to her need, it is not business as usual. You may encounter some resistance from your adult child. The pushback will be more severe in emotionally immature adult children, particularly if your previous approach was complete wish fulfillment.

ANTICIPATING LIKELY REACTIONS

You will, no doubt, hear some familiar refrains from your adult children if you don't respond favorably to their requests. All individuals deserve to be heard and active listening is essential to a productive relationship. But to avoid a repetition of old arguments, formulate your reactions and try some novel responses. Here are some examples:

- It isn't fair.
- I'll get in trouble if you don't _____.
- You're the only one who can help me.
- You helped my brother when he got into trouble.

He Says: It Isn't Fair

Thinking About Your Response:
When children are five or six, they often complain that "it isn't fair" if they don't get what they want when they want it. This regressed thinking needs to be abandoned by adults because frankly life isn't fair. People get injured in accidents and succumb to horrible diseases. These fates are random and "unfair." However, it is *not* unfair to refuse your adult child money, the chance to live at your home, or the right to use your car. Inform your child that as his parent you are committed to his well-being, but there is space between you and it's important for healthy adults to recognize that boundary.

He Says: I'll Get in Trouble If You Don't Get Me Out of This Mess

Thinking About Your Response:
No parent wants his child to return to jail because of an outstanding fine or face violence because of an unpaid street loan. For this reason you might choose to help in this crisis, but you must communicate that you didn't cause the problem and it is not your responsibility to fix it. If you perpetuate the

premise that you are always there to save him, he will surely repeat his mistakes. It's important for your child to hear from your mouth that the rules of engagement have changed.

There might be another situation that arises that does not carry immediate or dire consequences. Your child might need money for a superfluous purchase or another impulsive decision. In that circumstance, prove your point and do not reward self-defeating behavior.

She Says: You're the Only Person Who Can Help Me

Thinking About Your Response:

If you hear that you are the only person who can help, it's more likely that she means that you are the only person who *will* help her. Amy's daughter repeatedly turned to her in crisis. Amy says, "One of the hardest things I did was say no when she was in trouble but not in crisis. I saved her many times but most recently I resisted and she had no other choice but to pawn some of her special jewelry. I think this had an impact on her."

He Says: You Helped My Brother When *He* Got into Trouble

Thinking About Your Response:

Siblings constantly measure if they are getting their share of your attention and resources and this ad hoc accounting does not end in adulthood. Assume that you did help another adult child with a financial problem recently.

It's best to deal with this emotional blackmail quickly and honestly. Do not badmouth the other child. The amount may have been small and perhaps completely unsolicited. It may have gone to a child who rarely requests help. You only must reveal the details of the transaction that suit you and you cannot let their objection alter your course. What you and your spouse do with your money is no one else's business. Simply declare that you will not discuss the issue any further.

STANDING FIRM WITH YOUR PARTNER

Spouses and partners who work well together will be further challenged by the pressure of coping with a troubled adult child. You will need to fortify each other. No matter how dedicated you are to your child, your spouse is the vital person of your later life. A child might identify one of his parents as the softer target and will approach her repeatedly until he gets the answer he seeks. The job of the other spouse is to be supportive and to help her stand firm against the onslaught. The couple may need to stop speaking to their child for a while until the assault passes.

A unified approach is essential if your partner is not the child's biological parent. He may develop sympathy for your child, an interesting development if it happens. It is more likely, however, that he will take a harder line. It is easy to fall into the trap of confiding to the nonbiological parent that you are now adopting new tactics only to fall back to your previous ways. Don't allow such a situation to develop. Instead, if you don't agree with each other, then agree to disagree on this issue.

KEY POINTS IN THIS CHAPTER

- Try collaborating with your child to form a plan to resolve their most serious issues.

- Adult children often act in predictable ways when you refuse them what they want.

- If you say "no" to your child for a reason that is good enough for you, then stick with it in face of arguments.

- Work together with your spouse or partner (if you have one) to present a united front to your adult child.

CHAPTER 12
FACING REALITY
AND WALKING AWAY

We have not spoken to our son in months. He is addicted to pain medications. In the beginning, we tried everything to help him. We found him a job, and then he did not show up for work. We offered him money, and he squandered it. We gave him three chances at rehab, but he never took the programs seriously. We then decided that by helping him this way, we were actually hurting him. We finally stopped paying his rent. We stopped responding to his calls and e-mails, we changed the locks on our doors, and we told him not to contact us.

My husband really struggles with the lack of contact, and I know he has second thoughts. I actually am fairly calm. I might see my son at a family function or hear some gossip about him, but in truth I'm relieved that I don't know what is going on from moment to moment. But for my husband, it's like the sun went out.

Most of this book underlines available hope for your troubled adult child. Earlier chapters inform you about the relationship between mental illness and substance abuse and problematic behavior, and you learn that medications and proper psychotherapeutic techniques can dramatically improve even bleak situations. Helping troubled adult children is a marathon ordeal and efforts may need to be focused on seeking long-term relief like Social Security disability and Medicaid. Later chapters promote both understanding and managing the delicate relationships between your family members and friends in order to minimize the overall suffering associated with parenting a challenging adult child.

While the involvement of parents is essential to the recovery of many troubled adult children, sometimes even heroic efforts do not work. Some parents will come to the realization that the warm and positive relationship that they aspire to have is elusive and may not be possible. In these circumstances, a decision to withdraw from your child's life may be a rational step.

You may awaken one morning with the epiphany that all your efforts to help your child have been futile or, as is more likely, it might take years for you to conclude that you need an entirely new approach. The new strategy can be implemented in gradations, ranging from withdrawing financial resources to pursuing complete estrangement. However you arrive at this decision, you will inevitably feel cheated, sad, and perhaps relieved, and all at the same time. We hope the suggestions proposed earlier in the book prevent this standoff, but if this decision needs to be made, you need to be prepared.

WHY YOUR CHILD BREAKS YOUR HEART

Throughout this book, you've learned about why some adults are so difficult to parent. In general, troubled adult children fall into one of three categories: mental illness, personality disorders, and substance abuse disorders. Each has a different outcome and it is useful to see if your child falls into one of these categories. This will allow you to ascertain if your efforts will be productive.

Mental illnesses such as depression, psychosis, and ADHD explain many of the struggles of adult children. Very often, treating these biological illnesses greatly reduces the problems that have been created by your child's illness. A sneaky characteristic of many mental illnesses is a lack of insight: A person with active symptoms may not have the capacity to self-observe, for instance a person with bipolar mania is often the last to know that her behavior is off; it is often left to his parents to act on his behalf. Parents should be encouraged to help their children gain access to meaningful and effective treatments.

The prognosis is less favorable if you have an adult child with a personality disorder. Individuals in these groups do not seem to care how their behavior affects others. Adults with severe borderline personality disorder lack the capacity to sustain meaningful relationships and often fail miserably when they have their own children. Research into these personality disorders might eventually reveal that there is a biological underpinning to these behaviors. But in general, doctors apply these terms to individuals whose behavior cannot be explained by chemical imbalances. They respond less well to medications and traditional psychotherapy. They are often called criminals, not patients.

People with substance use disorders occupy the middle ground. This large heterogeneous group represents individuals suffering from alcohol or drug dependence. Their prognosis is highly variable. Some can spontaneously become clean and sober. Others need to work twelve-step programs to achieve success. If a patient with a substance use disorder has a treatable psychiatric condition like anxiety or ADHD, then treating the psychiatric condition can improve the chances of substance abuse recovery. On the other hand, a combination of opiate dependency and a severe personality disorder does not portend a good outcome.

Although your child probably falls into one of these disparate groups, it is not possible to absolutely predict how a particular individual will fare over time. And no matter their diagnosis, parents want to ensure that their children are managing their activities of daily living. Hopefully this includes getting an education, covering their rent and food, and maintaining productive relationships with others.

WHEN HELPING IS HURTING AND NOT HELPING IS HELPING

When does helping become counterproductive? Assisting your adult child by offering money or getting the most expensive criminal lawyer certainly curtails short-term crises, but it risks long-term problems. By taking such actions, you ensure that his dependency on you grows and suffocates the competing developmental process of separating from you. If your son is choosing to avoid personal responsibility, then paying his rent every month relieves his incentive to earn money. Why would he get a routine oil change if he knows that you would replace his cracked engine block? Softening every encounter with a creditor or probation officer certainly perpetuates his sense of incompetence.

Parents are not immortal, and all eventually become infirm and die. Whether they are Eagle Scouts or ex-cons, preparing your children for life after you are gone is a fundamental goal of parenting. You might not like the way they solve their problems—they may rent an apartment in an undesirable neighborhood or find a job that engenders considerable risk—but such steps must be viewed as the first steps toward independence.

To this end, there comes a time when withdrawing support is a reasonable tactic because it forces your adult child to address real life in real time. The degree to which you withdraw your support might depend on your child's diagnosis and prognosis. In some cases you might want to limit your financial contribution; in other circumstances you may choose to have more limited overall contact. This chapter describes parents who for various reasons have had to sever their relationship with their adult child altogether. Estrangement opens the door to the most intense emotions.

PULLING BACK

Gary relates the following story about his forty-year-old daughter Meredith, who has bipolar disorder. He says that she usually functions well or at least okay, and she and her husband live in a nice house that they own with their two children, ages ten and twelve. Her husband is a devoted father and has been a good husband.

Here's the problem: Three times in the past five years, Meredith has stopped taking her medications for bipolar disorder and has experienced major manic episodes. Each one was worse than the one before. The last time it happened, Meredith went without sleep for ten days. She got into a fight with her son's teacher that she likely instigated, and later in the day, Meredith was arrested for drunk driving. Shortly thereafter, Meredith gambled away most of the family savings at the downtown casino.

A pattern has developed. Each time when these episodes occur, Meredith's husband becomes so angry with her (and with reason) that he leaves. Unfortunately, he also leaves the children behind. Meredith's father said, "Then we start to fix the mess. My wife and I move in with our grandchildren, we get the kids to school and also get our daughter back on medications. We got Meredith a lawyer and set up a payment plan for her debt. After the start of each incident, in several weeks, she starts to get better and then our son-in-law comes around. We exit stage left and then everyone moves on. We never really talk about it because it's so painful."

The temptation for Meredith's father and his wife to intervene is clear. Their daughter has a treatable illness that predictably improves with time and taking her medication. Their grandchildren are at serious emotional risk when both parents go AWOL, and Meredith's father and mother have the financial resources and personal resourcefulness to solve the problems that his daughter creates.

But this time, Meredith's parents have decided on another course altogether. They want to get off this merry-go-round cycle. Gary says, "Going to the rescue on demand—and we never know when it will happen again—is too much for us to handle anymore. We will always protect our grandchildren, but we sat down with our daughter and her husband and told them that they need to step up and solve the problem on their own. Meredith needs to stay on her medication, and our son-in-law can no longer rely upon us to fill in for him in nearly every way, when he walks away from the problem. We are very sympathetic that our daughter has bipolar disorder, but they both need to take responsibility rather than shove it off on us. They also need to assume responsibility for their debt and solve their own financial problems. We are not responsible for her illness or their marriage. We are done."

SETTING LIMITS

Each family sets their own limits. For many years, Heather and Anna provided shelter to their son, Jake, an unemployed twenty-four-year-old man who was the product of Heather's first marriage. Heather and Anna were exasperated that Jake smoked marijuana daily and had periodic alcohol binges. When he smoked, he became passive and extremely unmotivated. When he drank he became mean and aggressive. Several times over the years, the police were called to the house and Jake was arrested for disturbing the peace. Neither his parents' pleading nor the humiliation of being led away in handcuffs in front of the neighbors changed Jake's recurrent behaviors.

Heather and Anna increasingly fought with each other about what to do with their son. Anna believed that tough love was the proper approach, and she said, "If we coddle him forever, he will never do anything for himself."

But Heather could not bring herself to throw Jake out, and said, "I can't do that to him. I would never forgive myself." After several months of counseling, they agreed on an intermediate step. Heather and Anna would insist that Jake leave their house, but they would help him pay for an apartment close by. They agreed to limit their contact to monthly visits.

The partial estrangement had mixed results. Living apart, Jake had less supervision and his substance use remained excessive. He was forced to find a job and although too much of his paycheck went to buying pot, he was functioning at a higher level. His absence from their home dialed down the chaos between Heather and Anna. The outcome was not ideal but it represented a positive step forward for the family.

WHEN TO CONSIDER ESTRANGEMENT

Partial steps may not be sufficient and more dramatic steps may be needed. A tactic of complete estrangement can be part of an active strategy to motivate your child to change. It can also be an act of default when there are no other options left for you to play. Either way, the decision to disengage from your adult child is a major life event and can occur for a number of reasons:

- Nothing you have tried works.
- His actions are appalling.
- The adult child's presence dooms the family.
- Your safety is in peril.

Nothing You Have Tried Works

Estrangement may be an option if there are no further options to help your adult child. A mother described her decision to cut off all contact with her adult son, saying, "Nothing worked for him. He smoked marijuana all day long, and he drank most nights. He was arrested four times in the past two years, and his legal fees were enormous. He would never consider getting treatment, because he really doesn't think he has a problem. For years, we tried to get him to go to treatment and we insisted that he go to Alcoholics Anonymous. At one point, the county sent him to court-ordered boot camp. Nothing worked. Finally we said, okay, go do it all by yourself. It has been eighteen months now, and my husband and I are actually doing okay with it. I'm surprised."

His Actions Are Appalling

For every crime, there is a perpetrator and nearly every perpetrator has a family. Families of criminals are more likely to become estranged from the offender. Mort and Lillian cut off contact with their son Rick after he was convicted of raping and murdering a college student. "We were devastated beyond belief, shamed, and angry," Lillian reports. "I was molested when I was a girl and I cannot fathom that my son could do something even worse."

Although ten years have passed and Lillian has made it clear that she has no intention of changing her position, not everyone in the family holds to the estrangement. Rick receives periodic visits from his older brother and sister, and his first cousin is helping him with an ongoing legal appeal. Somehow the family still functions by respecting each other's limits.

The Adult Child's Presence Dooms the Family

The decision to disengage is not always one that is chosen by the parents. Sometimes the child initiates the process or imposes unacceptable conditions for reconciliation. Estrangement is not always your own choice.

One mother, Geneva, described her daughter, Bonnie, who stopped contacting her and her husband three years ago. Geneva explains: "Bonnie started psychotherapy several years ago, at my suggestion. Within a few months, she became angry and distant and her therapist arranged a family meeting. It was actually a confrontation. At the meeting, Bonnie announced that my husband, her stepfather, had abused her as a child.

She said that the assaults began as a toddler and continued until she was age eleven. When I asked her why she did not tell me earlier, she said that I would not have believed her. Maybe she is right about that. When I suggested that there was a mistake, that the abuse was exaggerated, she told me that I was in denial and that my husband controls me."

Geneva's husband swears that the abuse did not happen. Geneva says, "For the life of me, I believe him. I have been with him for twenty-five years, we have a child together, and I know that he is not a pedophile. I can't imagine that he would do anything to hurt a child, let alone my child."

Geneva explains the rift in the family. Bonnie's oldest sister did not believe the claim, and said, "Bonnie is vulnerable and the therapist put her up to this. I was there and the abuse never happened." Bonnie's younger brother supported his sister and another child had no opinion.

"I am in a terrible bind," Geneva explains, "Bonnie insists that if I want to have any relationship with her, then I cannot stay with my husband. This also means that if I stand by him, I lose her."

In the end, Geneva did not agree to her daughter's conditions. She believed that she would have known if abuse occurred in her own home. She reasoned that other children would have direct knowledge of any abuse and they did not. In her heart she did not feel that her husband was culpable. She also knew that she might have been wrong. Their estrangement lasted several painful years.

Your Own Safety Is in Peril

Estrangement can also result from fear. All relationships are fueled by mutual trust. Once that is broken, and there are many degrees of betrayal, the future of the relationship is jeopardized. The following is a case of a family who cut off contact with their daughter because they felt that whatever good they could do for her was dwarfed by the threat of provoking her.

Carole says that her daughter made a death threat against her and her husband. Carole says, "I saw her note. She arranged for a friend of her then-boyfriend to kill us. At the time, she was beneficiary of our insurance policy. We don't think it was just a lark; she can be very cold-hearted and ruthless.

When she feels wronged, we are often the target of her rage. She migrates to evil boyfriends and the bad influence flows both ways. We have lost all trust in her. We have been estranged for about five years now. I pray for her because her life is constant chaos. But I know that we did the right thing."

COMMON EMOTIONS AFTER ESTRANGEMENT OCCURS

Many parents who feel that they must cast off their adult children in order to survive feel common emotions, such as the following feelings:

- Was it my fault?
- Will I ever see her again?
- What should I tell other people?
- How can I deal with this emotional pain?

Was It My Fault?

When their children's problems are first identified, nearly all parents blame themselves. Such emotions may resurface yet again when an estrangement occurs, even if parents cannot identify what they could have done differently to achieve a better outcome. Certain truths apply. The past cannot be changed, but it is helpful to discuss the past and your pain in a safe therapeutic setting. Very often the cause of estrangement is beyond our control. We cannot control our children—it's hard enough to control ourselves.

Most parents cut off contact with their children only after a long struggle and giving it the best they had. The challenge of therapy is to remain open to ideas about how you could have done better. This will help you with your other relationships and maybe over time with your estranged child. For this reason the best advice to Bonnie's mother is not to take sides in the bitter conflict but to be open to both parties. Time might clarify the past.

Will I Ever See Her Again?

The vast majority of parent-child estrangements do eventually end with reconciliation. But no one truly knows if this will ever happen or how long the freeze will last. The lack of contact with your adult child can be excruciating and painful. Endless nights might lie ahead wondering about what happens if he becomes sick or homeless. The agony of not knowing what is happening with your child is one of the most unappealing and dreadful aspects of parent-imposed estrangement.

At the same time, you should remember that you are imposing the estrangement not to punish your child, but because you need things to change. Estrangement becomes the weapon of last resort in this challenging relationship. Make it clear that you wish your child the best, and that you also hope that he receives treatment for substance abuse or a psychiatric condition before he ends up in prison or worse. The unsubtle message of estrangement is that you make it clear to your child that unless you do the right thing, then you cannot be in my life. If your child can make these changes, the possibility for reconciliation may remain open.

What Should We Tell Other People?

How many of the details of your family life should you disclose to friends and family? When there is estrangement with a child, parents need to take a unified approach over how they will handle the sensitive issue outside the home. The proper level of disclosure balances the parents' need for support with how carefully they want to protect their child's privacy.

Alex was a pathological liar and cocaine-dependent. His mother Claire felt that their decision to separate from their antisocial son was "not worth getting into with our friends and family. I was too mortified to tell the truth but I did not want to lie." In the first six months after Alex left home, Claire only knew that he was living in Florida. "When people asked me about him, I just said he was studying down south. It worked for me for a while."

Over the next several months, Claire grew more confident with her decision and was surprised to find comfort discussing the estrangement with sympathetic friends. A few family members offered unsolicited advice urging her to reconcile with Alex, but she felt empowered to shut them out. "I was uncomfortable with their opinions and we chose not to include them in my circle of support."

While Claire's approach evolved, her husband was more circumspect. Allen was a private and proud man, and he felt that Alex's situation should not be discussed freely. He reminded Claire that friends can change over a lifetime and not all are discreet. He told his wife, "There are no secrets. If you tell a few people about our son's problems—many others will soon know." Allen was irate with his son's antisocial behavior, but he was still protective of him. "It's not up to me to rat on Alex to others. He can lose his reputation only once. It's for him, not us, to decide what others will think of him."

How Can I Deal With This Emotional Pain?

Parents of troubled adult children are no strangers to emotional pain, and estrangement intensifies the sensation. This distress can feel like physical pain; stomach upset, headaches, and fatigue are common. (Read more about psychological and physical symptoms in chapter 9.) A certain amount of these symptoms is to be expected during the early stressful stages of estrangement.

If your anxiety and depression symptoms persist for more than four weeks or start to interfere with your daily life, then you might need to consult with a psychiatrist. Antidepressant and anti-anxiety medications can dampen these symptoms so that you can move on with your life. Ideally, your psychiatrist will also offer you counseling or arrange for you to see a therapist.

VULNERABLE TIMES AFTER AN ESTRANGEMENT

Just as mourners work through their stages of grief, the raw wound of estrangement eventually begins to heal. The day will come after you have not seen your adult child for months or even years and you are at peace with your decision to estrange. The sharp emotional pain that accompanied the initial period is replaced by something less intense. You become more comfortable alone in your thoughts.

Even when you have made progress, there are certain to be vulnerable moments. Your emotions may tug at you on your child's birthday, Christmas, or New Year's Eve. Happier times will be bittersweet memories. Be prepared that you are likely to feel bereaved at these special times and your resolve may be weakened. You will have to remind yourself that you cannot deal with your adult child as he is right now. The memories are real but they are far from the cold reality that compelled you to shut down the relationship.

RECONCILIATION: IS IT POSSIBLE?

There are no rules detailing the duration of estrangement. Estrangement can last weeks, months, or years. Tragically, some last forever.

At some point you will question whether it is time to take the first steps toward reconciliation. Estrangement is a dynamic process, affected by changing circumstances and the march of time. Ideally estrangement is not pursued as a punishment, rather as a means to encourage change. If you have evidence that your child has made changes, then it may be time to test the waters.

During the period of physical estrangement, some families let their child know the terms for re-engagement. At some point, your adult child may reestablish contact with you and may seem to genuinely want reconciliation. The parable of the Prodigal Son, who squandered his inheritance and returns home destitute into the arms of a forgiving father, gets replayed in families coping with estrangement.

Next Steps
Proceed with caution. The problem with initiating reconciliation is that you can appear overly anxious and your child can misinterpret your generous overture as a weakness. Make sure he knows that reconciliation is not an invitation for old habits to revisit. He cannot return to old patterns of handouts and deception. If your child initiates the contact, she should expect at a minimum to receive your healthy skepticism.

Questions to Ask Your Child
The true questions are whether she has really changed. Does she want forgiveness? Does she intend to chart a different course? Question her

carefully and listen intently. For example, if she says she is no longer abusing drugs, congratulate her and ask her how she overcame her addiction. It is a red flag if she claims she quit without help. Most substance abusers cannot simply stop using alcohol or drugs. Severely addicted individuals usually need to attend Alcoholics Anonymous or Narcotics Anonymous meetings at a minimum. Don't call her a liar but do keep your guard up. You can always insist that she prove her abstinence with random drug tests.

Ask open-ended questions that cannot be easily answered with a yes or no, so that the information that you receive will be more revealing. If the contact is made by telephone, you lose the information garnered by physical inspection. If the contact is made directly, and he shows up at your door disheveled and dirty, it's clear that he still has problems to resolve. Here are some examples of questions you may wish to ask:

- What have you been doing since we last had contact? (This may elicit a detailed answer. If he says, "Not much," then gently prod with, "Over all this time? Something must have happened!" Then listen for the answers.)

- Are you living nearby? (It's a good idea to discover where he is now, at least, in which state.)

- Have you seen any of your old friends? (His old friends may be directly connected with many of his old problems, such as substance abuse or criminal acts.)

If You Consider Reconciliation

Parental love can be very forgiving, and every parent hopes their child will grow and succeed. Still, do not lose sight of the tremendous emotional investment that you have made during the estrangement. Losing contact with your child involves self-doubt and many sleepless nights. Don't squander the investment with a rash and impulsive decision. The period of estrangement signifies that future proceedings will be different. Reconcile only after you are sure that your adult child is committed to change and wants you to help him change. Accept the request only if you are committed to the boundaries you have established.

Granted, you might make the wrong choice. The same problems that led to your estrangement might soon reappear and the reconciliation may be short-lived. If this does happen, then be confident that you have sent the strongest message in the service of your child's recovery. Hearts can be rebroken. Sometimes the risk is worth taking.

KEY POINTS IN THIS CHAPTER

- Sometimes you need to consider breaking off your relationship with your adult child.
- Certain times can make the estrangement very hard, such as your birthday, the child's birthday, or the holidays.
- Common emotions experienced after an estrangement are fear that you may never see your child again or wondering how you can manage your emotional pain.
- Reconciliation is possible after estrangement—but go slowly.

CONCLUSION

How does your adult child break your heart? Let us count the ways. Does he not work? Does she steal from local businessmen? Does he father children and not support them? The human drama is written in a binary language. There are criminals and there are victims, those who shoot and those who get shot, those who exploit the system and those who pay their taxes.

The mentally ill, substance abusers, criminals, and freeloaders walk alongside us and they do not find many sympathetic audiences. They are usually pegged on the dark side of the right versus wrong calculation. But they are our fellow creatures, they have families and partners who love them, and they have suffering parents.

Each day, we are all exposed to the litany of crime and punishment that dominates the news. We quiver at the tragedies and feel fortunate that our child was not a passenger in the car that crashed the night before. We rejoice that it was not our grandchildren who were stranded in the house that burned to the ground. We think about the family of today's victim and imagine their horror.

Parents of troubled adults watch the same news, yet they absorb it with a different sensibility. They know it could have been their drunken son barreling into the group of kids. It could have been their daughter passed out from drugs in the burning house while her kids slept unsuspectingly in the room above. Parents of troubled adult children turn up the radio and listen intently for details. A relief. Not my child. Not our family. Not this time. They exhale. This day has passed.

The words of a book are intended to be read for years but are shaped by the moments in which they are written. These chapters were written through the near fatal shooting of an Arizona congresswoman, the theater massacre at a midnight movie in Colorado, and the unfathomable murder of first graders and their teachers in Newtown, Connecticut. Like the rest of the nation, we watched the manhunt for two Chechen brothers who left pressure bombs at the feet of spectators at the 2013 Boston Marathon. As we wrote, we knew that these headlines would soon be replaced by others. We thought about the mothers and fathers and brothers and sisters of those touched by these events.

Recently I met with a patient whom I had not seen in a couple of months. In an earlier chapter I wrote a portion of his daughter's story. After years of drug abuse, she had left home without a trail, lured by an irresponsible boyfriend who promised her great adventure. She was found by a private investigator a year later dancing in a lonely nightclub outside Las Vegas. At our last meeting my patient was so happy that his daughter was home. That was my last update.

"How have things been?" I asked.

He looked grim. "She did not do well after she came home. She was weak and I took her to the doctor. She was diagnosed with HIV. She wanted no part of AIDS treatment and within a couple weeks, she went back west. She continued to drink and use meth. We've had no contact."

He continued, "We just got a call from the public defender. She was arrested for filming a sex scene in public. At first they wrote her up for indecent exposure. Today they added the charge of willfully transmitting a communicable disease. It's a felony, but I think she will die before they try her."

My usual reservoir of comforting words failed me. I changed the subject to more comfortable ground.

"You know I'm writing a book on raising troubled adult children."

"Oh yeah. How does it end?"

Pointed questions demand good answers. Here's the truth. It ends up differently for every family. The last twelve chapters are an attempt to organize this enormous topic. We have observed the challenges of raising troubled adult children and the specific problems that occur when they live under your roof. We discussed the sense of shame that some parents feel over this troubled relationship. We explored mental health and the courts and proposed some ways for families to negotiate their way through the criminal justice system. We defined the major mental illnesses that occur in young adults and the medications used to treat them.

These conditions scar families forever, a pain surpassed only by parents touched by a child's suicide.

The toll of parenting a troubled adult child is never fully paid. During this struggle, parents need to promote their own physical and mental health and preserve their relationships with friends and other family members. They must take creative approaches to help their child solve problems and recognize when the struggle is over and there is no more that can be done.

So how does it end? Some families are lucky—some are not. Some adult children learn from the past—others are intractable. The central theme of this book is that mental illness and substance use disorders are at the core of many troubled adult children. Parents must do what they can and take control of as much as possible. Do your best to ensure that your child gets aggressive mental health treatment.

We end our book by noting some positive developments and some concerning trends. In 2014, the Affordable Care Act will be fully instituted. More Americans than ever will have health care insurance. Already this legislation has allowed children up to age twenty-six to remain under their parents' insurance. Mental health benefits are approaching parity with other medical conditions, and while coverage remains imperfect, it is better than in past decades. The political parties will continue to debate this reform, and by offering more we should not retreat from existing commitments. Overall, families of troubled adults will benefit as more coverage is extended.

Mental illness is still stigmatized in the public square. Addiction should be viewed as a health problem, not a criminal problem, and progress on this front is slow. Still, more and more people are talking about their struggles with anxiety and depression and substance abuse. There is a greater public awareness of autism. America is growing more comfortable with these topics.

There is also a better understanding of brain-based illnesses. In the next decade, the federal Brain Research through Advancing Innovative Neurotechnologies (BRAIN) initiative will map the activities of individual cells and neurons. More Americans are getting treated for anxiety, depression, and ADHD and treatments are getting better.

Of concern, there is a nationwide shortage of psychiatrists. In some cities and rural areas, the mentally ill can barely get in to see their doctors. Physician extenders like psychiatric nurse practitioners and physician assistants have begun to play a vital role in health care delivery. Alarmingly, the American pharmaceutical industry has been vilified and many obstacles block the development of successful medications. Several major drug developers have pulled up stakes due to the long odds of bringing new psychiatric treatments to market. The number of treatments approved each year by the FDA has decreased markedly compared to the productive years of the 1990s.

Some of these issues are reversible and will change with shifting political sands. The concerns of parents of troubled children however are timeless. They will always need knowledge and hope and the support of their community to mend their broken hearts. We hope this book has made inroads into this larger mission.

ACKNOWLEDGMENTS

Special thanks from both authors to Randi Kreger for facilitating key research in our book. Randi placed a notice on her blog (bpdcentral.com) asking parents of troubled adult children to respond to our questionnaire, and Kreger also told others on related blogs about the questionnaire. Hundreds responded and were very candid about their struggles with their adult children. Parents who responded to the questionnaire had adult children with many different disorders, including bipolar disorder, borderline personality disorder, major depression, and psychotic disorders. Kreger is the author of excellent books on borderline personality disorder, including *The Essential Family Guide to Borderline Personality Disorder: New Tools and Techniques to Stop Walking on Eggshells* (Hazelden, 2008) and *Stop Walking on Eggshells: Taking Your Life Back When Someone You Care About Has Borderline Personality Disorder*, Second Edition (New Harbinger Publications, 2010).

Thanks also to Canadian academic Anne-Marie Ambert for her book emphasizing the effect of children on parents of all ages: *The Effect of Children on Parents*, Second Edition (Haworth Press, 2001), and also for her encouragement with pursuing our book.

Both authors wish to thank the survey respondents, whose comments and deep suffering are illustrated throughout this book by their quotations. These comments have been edited only slightly for grammar and clarity and to conceal the respondents' identity.

Last, both authors wish to thank editors Mary Norris and Tracee Williams for their excellent recommendations, which considerably improved our book.

JOEL L. YOUNG, MD

My coauthor Christine Adamec developed the idea of writing a book for parents of troubled adult children. Her ability to organize vast material and her optimistic adherence to the schedule were vital to our project.

I thank my children—Benjamin, Katie, and Emily—for their support. I recall most fondly the times when they did their own work alongside me. My wife, Mindy Layne Young, JD, MSW, accepted the sacrifices needed to complete this book and offered her valuable professional insight. Finally, I am indebted to my patients and their families who entrust me to offer care and counsel during critical times. With this book, I am hopeful that our shared experiences will offer guidance to other parents facing similar struggles.

CHRISTINE ADAMEC

I would like to thank my loving family for their continued support through the course of the three years that were spent on researching and writing this book with Dr. Young.

APPENDICES

For individuals who need further information, Appendix A lists contact information for important national organizations, Appendix B includes a variety of informative websites, and Appendix C lists child abuse hotlines to call if you know or suspect that your adult child or someone else is abusing or neglecting their children.

APPENDIX A

IMPORTANT NATIONAL ORGANIZATIONS THAT MAY HELP

Note: The authors do not endorse any of these organizations and provide their addresses and phone numbers for information only.

Alcoholics Anonymous World
   Services
475 Riverside Drive at West 120th
   Street, 11th Floor
New York, NY 10115
(212) 870-3400
www.aa.org

American Psychological
   Association
750 First Street NE
Washington, DC 20002-4242
(800) 374-2721
(202) 336-5500
www.apa.org

American Psychiatric Association
1000 Wilson Boulevard, Suite 1825
Arlington, VA 22209
(888) 357-7924 or (888) 35-PSYCH
www.psych.org

Anxiety and Depression Association of America
8701 Georgia Avenue, #412
Silver Spring, MD 20910
(240) 485-1001
www.adaa.org

Children and Adults with
   Attention-Deficit/Hyperactivity
   Disorder
8181 Professional Place, Suite 150
Landover, MD 20785
(301) 306-7070
www.chadd.org

Families of Adults Affected by
   Asperger's Syndrome
FAAAS, Inc.
PO Box 514
Centerville, MA 02632
(508) 790-1930
faaas.org

Mothers of Incarcerated Sons
PO Box 401335
Redford, MI 48240
(248) 579-5469
www.mothersofinmates.org

National Alliance for Mental Illness (NAMI)
3803 N. Fairfax Drive, Suite 100
Arlington, VA 22203
(703) 524-7600
www.nami.org

National Institute on Drug Abuse
(NIDA)
Office of Science Policy and Communications, Public Information and Liaison Branch
6001 Executive Boulevard, Room
5213, MSC 9561
Bethesda, MD 20892-9561
(301) 443-1124
www.drugabuse.gov

National Institute of Mental Health
(NIMH)
Science Writing, Press, and Dis-
semination Branch
6001 Executive Boulevard, Room
6200, MSC 9663
Bethesda, MD 20892-9663
(866) 615-6464
www.nimh.nih.gov

Substance Abuse and Mental
Health Services Administration
SAMHSA's Health Information
Network
PO Box 2345
Rockville, MD 20847-2345
(877) 726-4727
www.samhsa.gov

KEY WEBSITES

Al-Anon/Alateen www.al-anon.alateen.org/how-to-find-a-meeting

Cocaine Anonymous World Services www.ca.org

Compassionate Friends www.compassionatefriends.org

Families Anonymous familiesanonymous.org

Heroin Anonymous World Services www.heroin-anonymous.org

International Bipolar Foundation www.internationalbipolarfoundation.org

International OCD Foundation www.ocfoundation.org

Marijuana Anonymous www.marijuana-anonymous.org

Narcotics Anonymous World Services www.na.org

Pills Anonymous World Services www.pillsanonymous.org

Women for Sobriety womenforsobriety.org

Women's Health www.womenshealth.gov/mental-health/your-rights/americans-disability-act.cfm

STATE-BY-STATE LISTING OF CHILD ABUSE HOTLINES

If you have a valid reason to believe that your grandchild or another child is being abused or neglected, or is in serious danger of abuse or neglect (for example, because the suspected perpetrator is a drug abuser, alcoholic, or a mentally ill person off his medications), and you have also seen evidence of possible or likely abuse, then you should contact the state protective services hotline. This appendix provides a state-by-state listing. You may also wish to contact local police. A child's life is more important than any embarrassment you may feel or any negative feelings your adult child may harbor against you, should they discover that you made the call. These numbers are current as of July 29, 2013.

Note: Some numbers provide the phone number of Childhelp, an organization that will give further information on how to report abuse or neglect, while many states have their own number to call.

Alabama
(334) 242-9500

Alaska
(800) 478-4444

Arizona
(888) 767-2445

Arkansas
(800) 482-5964

California
(800) 422-4453

Colorado
(303) 866-5932

Connecticut
(800) 842-2288

Delaware
(800) 292-9582

District of Columbia
(202) 671-7233

Florida
(800) 962-2873

Georgia
(800) 422-4453

Hawaii
(800) 832-5300

Idaho
(800) 926-2588

Illinois
(800) 252-2873

Indiana
(800) 800-5556

Iowa
(800) 362-2178

Kansas
(800) 922-5330

Kentucky
(877) 597-2331

Louisiana
(855) 452-5437

Maine
(800) 963-9490

Maryland
(800) 422-4453

Massachusetts
(800) 792-5200

Michigan
(855) 444-3911

Minnesota
(800) 422-4453

Mississippi
(800) 222-8000

Missouri
(800) 392-3738

Montana
(866) 820-5437

Nebraska
(800) 652-1999

Nevada
(800) 992-5757

New Hampshire
(800) 894-5533

New Jersey
(877) 652-2873

New Mexico
(855) 333-7233

New York
(800) 342-3720

North Carolina
(800) 422-4453

North Dakota
(800) 422-4453

Ohio
(800) 642-4453

Oklahoma
(800) 522-3511

Oregon
(800) 422-4453

Pennsylvania
(800) 932-0313

Puerto Rico
(800) 981-8333

Rhode Island
(800) 742-4453

South Carolina
(803) 898-7318

South Dakota
(800) 422-4453

Tennessee
(877) 237-0004

Texas
(800) 252-5400

Utah
(800) 323-3237

Vermont
(800) 649-5285

Virginia
(800) 552-7096

Washington
(800) 562-5624

West Virginia
(800) 352-6513

Wisconsin
(800) 422-4453

Wyoming
(800) 422-4453

BIBLIOGRAPHY

Adamec, Christine. *How to Live with a Mentally Ill Person*. New York: Wiley, 1996.

Adamec, Christine. *Impulse Control Disorders*. New York: Chelsea House, 2008.

Adamec, Christine. *Opium*. New York: Chelsea House, 2014.

Ambert, Anne-Marie. *The Effect of Children on Parents*. Second Edition. New York: Haworth Press, 2001.

Aschbrenner, K. A., et al. "Subjective Burden and Personal Gains among Older Parents of Adults with Serious Mental Illness." *Psychiatric Services* 61, no. 6 (2010): 605–11.

Barak, D., and Z. Solomon. "In the Shadow of Schizophrenia: A Study of Siblings' Perceptions." *Israel Journal of Psychiatry and Related Sciences* 42, no. 4 (2005): 234–41.

Barbaresi, W. J., et al. "Mortality, ADHD, and Psychosocial Adversity in Adults with Childhood ADHD: A Prospective Study." *Pediatrics* (2013), pediatrics.aappublications.org/content/early/2013/02/26/peds.2012-2354.full.pdf+html, accessed April 5, 2013.

Bolton, James M., MD, et al. "Parents Bereaved by Offspring Suicide: A Population-Based Longitudinal Case-Control Study." *JAMA Psychiatry* 70, no. 2 (2012): 158–67.

Borges, Guilherme, et al. "Psychiatric Disorders, Comorbidity, and Suicidality in Mexico." *Journal of Affective Disorders* 124, nos. 1–2 (2010): 98–107.

Brown, Harriet. "Looking for Evidence That Therapy Works." *New York Times*, March 25, 2013, well.blogs.nytimes.com/2013/03/25/looking-for-evidence-that-therapy-works, accessed April 17, 2013.

Centers for Disease Control and Prevention. "Suicide: Facts at a Glance, 2012." 2012, www.cdc.gov/violenceprevention/pdf/suicide-datasheet-a.PDF, accessed January 30, 2013.

Clark, Robin E., PhD, Judith Freeman Clark with Christine Adamec. *The Encyclopedia of Child Abuse.* Third Edition. New York: Facts On File, 2007.

Cody, Mark A. "Heading in Opposite Directions—Two New Mental Laws." Michigan Protection & Advocacy Service. (undated). Available online at www.mpas.org/Article.asp?TOPIC=10944. Accessed June 2, 2013.

Copeland, Darcy A., and MarySue V. Heilemann. "Choosing 'The Best of the Hells': Mothers Face Housing Dilemmas for Their Adult Children with Mental Illness and a History of Violence." *Qualitative Health Research* 21, no. 4 (2011): 520–33.

Copello, Alex G., Richard D. B. Velleman, and Lorna J. Templeton. "Family Interventions in the Treatment of Alcohol and Drug Problems." *Drug and Alcohol Reviews* 24 (2005): 369–85.

Crary, David. "Those Who Survived Suicide Attempts Begin to Reach Out to Help Others." Associated Press, April 15, 2013, www.freep.com/article/20130415/NEWS07/304150025/Those-who-survived-suicide-attempts-begin-to-reach-out-to-help-others, accessed April 28, 2013.

Cross-Disorder Group of the Psychiatric Genomics Consortium. "Identification of Risk Loci with Shared Effects on Five Major Psychiatric Disorders: A Genome-Wide Analysis." *Lancet* 381 (April 20, 2013): 1371–1379.

Crump, Casey, et al. "Mental Disorders and Vulnerability to Homicidal Death: Swedish Nationwide Cohort Study." *British Medical Journal* 346 (2013), www.bmj.com/content/346/bmj.f557, accessed April 25, 2013.

Fazel, Seena, MD, et al. "Bipolar Disorder and Violent Crime: New Evidence from Population-Based Longitudinal Studies and Systematic Review." *Archives of General Psychiatry* 67, no. 9 (2010): 931–38.

Fingerman, Karen L., et al. "Only as Happy as the Least Happy Child: Multiple Grown Children's Problems and Successes and Middle-aged Parents' Well-being." *Journal of Gerontology,* Series B 67, no. 2 (2011): 184–93.

Forest Laboratories, Inc. "CAMPRAL Full Prescribing Information." www.frx.com/pi/campral_pi.pdf, accessed August 6, 2013.

George, David T., et al. "A Model Linking Biology, Behavior and Psychiatric Diagnoses in Perpetrators of Domestic Violence." *Medical Hypotheses* 67 (2006): 345–53.

Gold, Mark S., MD, and Christine Adamec. *The Encyclopedia of Alcoholism and Alcohol Abuse.* New York: Facts On File, 2010.

Grant, David, et al. "More Than Half a Million California Adults Seriously Thought about Suicide in the Past Month." *Health Policy Brief,* no volume, no number. December 2012, healthpolicy.ucla.edu/ publications/Documents/PDF/test1.pdf, accessed February 7, 2013.

Grohol, John. "15 Common Cognitive Distortions." *Psych Central,* 2009, psychcentral.com/lib/2009/15-common-cognitive-distortions, accessed April 15, 2013.

Hart, Christina, et al. "A UK Population-Based Study of the Relationship between Mental Disorder and Victimisation." *Social Psychiatry and Psychiatric Epidemiology* 47 (2012): 1581–90.

Hay, Elizabeth L., Karen L. Fingerman, and Eva S. Lefkowitz. "The Worries Adult Children and Their Parents Experience for One Another." *Aging and Human Development* 67, no. 2 (2008): 101–27.

Johansson, Anita, RN, et al. "Fathers' Everyday Experiences of Having an Adult Child Who Suffers from Long-Term Mental Illness." *Issues in Mental Health Nursing* 33 (2012): 109–17.

Jones, Lisa, et al. "Prevalence and Risk of Violence Against Children with Disabilities: A Systematic Review and Meta-analysis of Observational Studies." *Lancet* 380, no. 9845 (2012): 899–907.

Kahn, Joan R., Frances Goldscheider, and Javier Garcia-Manglano. "Growing Parental Economic Power in Parent-Adult Child Households: Coresidence and Financial Dependency in the United States, 1960–2010. *Demography* 50, no. 1 (2013).

Karp, David A. *The Burden of Sympathy: How Families Cope with Mental Illness.* New York: Oxford University Press, 2001.

Kasckow, John, Kandi Felmet, and Sidney Zisook. "Managing Suicide Risk in Patients with Schizophrenia." *CNS Drugs* 25, no. 2 (2011): 129–43.

Kolata, Gina. "5 Disorders Share Genetic Risk Factors, Study Finds." *New York Times*, February 28, 2013, www.nytimes.com/2013/03/01/health/study-finds-genetic-risk-factors-shared-by-5-psychiatric-disorders.html?_r=3&, accessed February 28, 2013.

Lamb, H. Richard, MD. "Meeting the Needs of Those Persons With Serious Mental Illness Who Are Most Likely to Become Criminalized." *Journal of the American Academy of Psychiatry and the Law* 39 (2011): 549–54.

Lamb, H. Richard, MD. "Reversing Criminalization." *American Journal of Psychiatry* 166, no. 1 (2009): 8–10.

Lichtenstein, Paul, et al. "Medication for Attention Deficit-Hyperactivity Disorder and Criminality." *New England Journal of Medicine* 367, no. 21 (November 22, 2012): 2006–14.

Long, Liza. "I Am Adam Lanza's Mother." *Blue Review*, Boise State University, December 15, 2012, thebluereview.org/i-am-adam-lanzas-mother, accessed February 15, 2013.

Manchikanti, Laxmaiah, MD, et al. "Opioid Epidemic in the United States." *Pain Physician* 15 (2012): ES9–ES39.

Mayo Clinic Staff. "Intervention: Help a Loved One Overcome Addiction." Mayo Clinic, August 23, 2011, www.mayoclinic.com/health/intervention/MH00127, accessed February 18, 2013.

Mazzone, Luigi, Liliana Ruta, and Laura Reale. "Psychiatric Comorbidities in Asperger's Syndrome and High Functioning Autism: Diagnostic Challenges." *Annals of General Psychiatry* 11, www.annals-general-psychiatry.com/content/11/1/16, accessed January 16, 2013.

National Institute of Mental Health. *Anxiety Disorders.* Bethesda, MD: US Department of Health and Human Services, 2009, www.nimh .nih.gov/health/publications/anxiety-disorders/nimhanxiety.pdf, accessed September 4, 2012.

National Institute of Mental Health. *Borderline Personality Disorder.* Undated. Bethesda, MD: US Department of Health and Human Services, www.nimh.nih.gov/health/publications/borderline-personality-disorder/borderline_personality_disorder_508.pdf, accessed September 4, 2012.

National Institute of Mental Health. *Obsessive-Compulsive Disorder: When Unwanted Thoughts Take Over.* Bethesda, MD: US Department of Health and Human Services, 2010, www.nimh.nih.gov/health/ publications/obsessive-compulsive-disorder-when-unwanted-thoughts-take-over/ocd-trifold.pdf, accessed January 19, 2013.

National Institute of Mental Health. "Suicide in the U.S.: Statistics and Prevention." Undated, www.nimh.nih.gov/health/publications/ suicide-in-the-us-statistics-and-prevention/index.shtml, accessed January 30, 2013.

National Institute of Mental Health. *Schizophrenia.* Bethesda, MD: US Department of Health and Human Services, 2009, www.nimh.nih .gov/health/publications/schizophrenia/schizophrenia-booket-2009.pdf, accessed November 13, 2012.

National Institute on Drug Abuse. *The Science of Addiction: Drugs, Brains, and Behavior.* Bethesda, MD: National Institutes of Health, April 2007, Revised August 2010, www.drugabuse.gov/sites/default/files/ sciofaddiction.pdf, accessed February 16, 2013.

National Library of Medicine. "Alcoholism and Alcohol Abuse." *A.D.A.M. Medical Encyclopedia,* March 20, 2011, www.ncbi.nlm.nih.gov/pubmed health/PMH0001940, accessed February 21, 2013.

Nock, M. K., et al. "Mental Disorders, Comorbidity and Suicidal Behavior: Results from the National Comorbidity Survey Replication." *Molecular Psychiatry* 15, no. 8 (2010): 868–76.

Richardson, Meg, et al. "Parents' Grief in the Context of Adult Child Mental Illness: A Qualitative Review." *Clinical Child and Family Psychology Review* 14 (2011): 28–43.

Smith, Judith R. "Listening to Older Adult Parents of Adult Children with Mental Illness." *Journal of Family Social Work* 15 (2012): 126–40.

Soloff, Paul H., MD, and Laurel Chiappetta. "Prospective Predictors of Suicidal Behavior in BPD at 6 Year Follow-up." *American Journal of Psychiatry* 199, no. 5 (2012): 484–90.

Spiegel, Alix. "More and More, Favored Psychotherapy Lets Bygones Be Bygones." *New York Times*, February 14, 2006, www.nytimes.com/2006/02/14/health/psychology/14psyc.html?pagewanted=all&_r=2&, accessed April 17, 2013.

Substance Abuse and Mental Health Services Administration. "8.6 Million Adults Had Suicidal Thoughts in the Past Year." *Data Spotlight*, September 10, 2012.

Substance Abuse and Mental Health Services Administration. "State Estimates of Nonmedical Use of Prescription Pain Relievers." *The NSDUH Report*, January 8, 2013.

Tondo, Leonardo, MD, and Ross J. Baldessarini, MD. "Can Suicide Be Prevented? The Role of Lithium and Other Psychotropics." *Psychiatric Times* 28, no. 2 (February 10, 2011), www.psychiatrictimes.com/bipolar-disorder/content/article/10168/1795342, accessed January 30, 2013.

Trevillion, Kylee, et al. "Experiences of Domestic Violence and Mental Disorders: A Systematic Review and Meta-Analysis." *PLOS One*, December 26, 2012, www.plosone.org/article/info%3Adoi%2F10.1371%2Fjournal.pone.0051740, accessed April 25, 2013.

US Department of Health and Human Services, Office of the Surgeon General, and National Action Alliance for Suicide Prevention. *2012 National Strategy for Suicide Prevention: Goals and Objectives for Action*. Washington, DC: US Department of Health and Human Services, September 2012.

US Department of Health and Human Services, Administration for Children and Families, Administration on Children, Youth, and Families, Children's Bureau. *Child Maltreatment 2011*. 2012, www.acf.hhs.gov/sites/default/files/cb/cm11.pdf, accessed February 25, 2013.

Van Dorn, Richard, Jan Volavka, and Norman Johnson. "Mental Disorder and Violence: Is There a Relationship Beyond Substance Use?" *Social Psychiatry and Psychiatric Epidemiology*, 2011, mentalillnesspolicy.org/consequences/mental-disorder-violence-2011.pdf, accessed April 24, 2013.

Wells, Kathryn, MD. "Substance Abuse and Child Maltreatment." *Pediatric Clinics of North America* 56 (2009): 345–62.

Wilens, Timothy E., MD, and Nicholas R. Morrison. "The Intersection of Attention-deficit/Hyperactivity Disorder and Substance Abuse." *Current Opinions in Psychiatry* 24, no. 4 (2011): 280–85.

Woodbury-Smith, Marc R., and Fred R. Volkmar. "Asperger's Syndrome." *European Child & Adolescent Psychiatry* 18, no. 1 (2008): 2–11.

Yip, Paul S. F., et al. "Means Restriction for Suicide Prevention." *Lancet* 379 (June 23, 2012): 2393–99.

Young, Joel, MD. *ADHD Grown Up: A Guide to Adolescent and Adult ADHD*. New York: W. W. Norton and Company, 2007.

Young, Joel, MD. *Contemporary Diagnosis and Management of Adult ADHD*. Longboat Key, FL: Handbooks in Health Care, 2009.

Zieve, David, MD, and David C. Dugdale III. "Alcoholism and Alcohol Abuse." March 20, 2011, www.ncbi.nlm.nih.gov/pubmedhealth/PMH0001940, accessed February 16, 2013.

Zieve, David, MD. "Opiate Withdrawal." MedlinePlus. National Institutes of Health. January 23, 2012. Available online at www.nlm.nih.gov/medlineplus/ency/article/000949.htm. Accessed June 2, 2013.

INDEX

246

ABOUT THE AUTHORS

Joel L. Young, MD is the founder and medical director of the Rochester Center for Behavioral Medicine in Rochester Hills, Michigan. Dr. Young obtained his medical degree from Wayne State University School of Medicine and then served as the Adult Service Chief Resident (Psychiatry) at the University of Michigan Hospitals. He is certified by the American Board of Psychiatry and Neurology, and holds added qualifications in forensic and geriatric psychiatry. In addition, he is a diplomate of the American Board of Adolescent Psychiatry. He is on staff at William Beaumont Hospital and teaches Wayne State University resident physicians.

Dr. Young has been a principal investigator in more than fifty-five clinical trials related to ADHD, bipolar disorder, depression, dementia, and eating disorders. He has published sixty articles and textbook chapters, and is a frequent contributor to Medscape and other online resources. His book, *ADHD Grown Up: A Guide to Adolescent and Adult ADHD* (W. W. Norton and Company), was published in 2007. His second book, *Contemporary Diagnosis and Management of Adult ADHD* (2009) was directed at specialty clinicians.

Young is a frequent source for writers and reporters exploring mental illness and the family. He and his clinic routinely advise parents of severely ill adult children on issues emanating from psychiatric illnesses, substance abuse, criminal behavior, and suicide.

Christine Adamec is a medical and self-help book writer who has written more than thirty books and encyclopedias for publishers such as Wiley, McGraw-Hill, and Facts On File. She also coauthored *The Encyclopedia of Kidney Diseases and Disorders* (Facts On File, 2011) and coauthored the popular *Fibromyalgia for Dummies* (Wiley, 2007), a book that has sold 100,000 copies in two editions. Adamec has also written or coauthored numerous books on substance abuse and dependence as well as mental illness, including *Opium* (Chelsea House, in press for 2014), *Amphetamines and Methamphetamine* (Chelsea House, 2011), *The Encyclopedia of Alcoholism and Alcohol Abuse* (Facts On File, 2010), and *How to Live with a Mentally Ill Person* (Wiley, 1996). Adamec is a member of the American Society of Journalists & Authors and the American Medical Writers Association.